WHAT IF WE STOP SAYING PLACEBO?

After Placebo

IN
MEDICAL RESEARCH
AND CLINICAL PRACTICE

Robin Nunn

ARJANA MEDIA

Published by Arjana Media
arjana.com/afterplacebo

After Placebo
in medical research and clinical practice

Library and Archives Canada Cataloguing in Publication

Nunn, Robin, author
    After placebo : in medical research and clinical practice / Robin Nunn.
    Includes bibliographical references.
    ISBN 978-0-9947316-1-6 (bound).--ISBN 978-0-9947316-0-9 (paperback)
        1. Placebos (Medicine). 2. Medicine--Research. I. Title.
        RM331.N85 2015   615.5   C2015-902330-0

First Arjana Edition
10 9 8 7 6 5 4 3 2 1

CONTENTS

Many thanks to Catherine Burwell, Iain Chalmers, Michael Cournoyea, Jennifer Decorte, Jackie Duffin, Murry Enkin, Ian Hacking, André Leblanc, Claire Letemendia, Mark Nunn, Leanne Schmidt, Kevin Thorpe, Andrew Turner and to those whose probing questions in my classes and presentations helped to improve this work.

1 Introduction

Placebo seems to be everywhere in medicine. Estimates of placebo use in clinical practice vary widely, partly because it's difficult to say what a placebo is, but there is general agreement that physicians commonly use the fake treatments they call placebos. Fake treatments are also a primary standard of comparison in clinical trials and have become central to experimental methodology in medical research. Consequently more experimental subjects have received placebo treatments than any single experimental treatment.

Placebo is so pervasive that it has been described as the one common element in all medical treatments in all of medical history (Shapiro and Shapiro 1997, Benedetti 2009). Placebos have been labeled as the "most adaptable, protean, effective, safe and cheap drugs in the world's pharmacopoeia" (Buckman and Sabbagh 1993). For common therapies that do not have large obvious effects, some researchers have gone so far as to view all therapy as placebo (Lindahl and Linwall 1982).

Yet no satisfactory account of placebo has been provided. No agreement has been reached on what placebo is, what effects it has or whether it even exists. The concept of placebo continues to perplex medical professionals, historians and philosophers. I think that the placebo concept itself is the problem.

Placebo is an unstable construct, not a stable phenomenon. Placebo talk conceals more than it reveals. The main thesis of the following discussion is that the placebo concept is so problematic that it should be abandoned. To summarize this work in one normative sentence:

> We should abandon the outdated notion of placebo and start thinking in terms that will improve medical research and clinical practice.

Or for the really short sound bite, here are six words that suggest we should begin now to imagine and create the future of medicine after placebo:

> What if we stop saying placebo?

The implications and opportunities in a post-placebo viewpoint for medicine and health are vast. We need new research literature, new textbooks, new training and new laws that expunge the notion of placebo or replace it with a clear admission that we just don't know, rather than continue to obfuscate in terms of placebo.

I began to envision medicine after placebo as part of a broader inquiry into sources of medical knowledge, and in particular while considering how we know what works in medicine. Possible sources of medical knowledge, among others, include relying on medical experts, adopting traditional folk practices, accepting the advice of celebrities and reading the medical literature.

Currently the most highly valued source of medical knowledge in Western biomedicine is not expertise, experience, tradition, fame or Doctor Google, but rather is the randomized placebo-controlled clinical trial that forms the core methodology of evidence-based medicine. Curiously, this clinical trial methodology that purports to bring scientific credibility to medical interventions rests on something mysterious, placebo and its effects, that nobody can sensibly define let alone fully understand.

If you already find placebo to be a confusing and mysterious notion, then maybe this discussion will give you more support in our mutual efforts to move medicine beyond placebo. If you're not ready to discard placebo yet, then I hope to change your mind in the sentences that follow. They set out many problems with the present placebo paradigm and indicate how medical research and clinical practice could benefit if the whole placebo notion were discarded. Putting medical research and clinical practice on a placebo-free, dichotomy-reduced diet, I outline what's wrong with saying placebo and what might be said after we agree that placebo is no longer the way to say it. This discussion goes beyond criticism of placebo to offer a constructive vision of the future.

A brief placebo history

At various times during its history, placebo has been everything from deceiver to pest to hero. As deceiver, placebo is mock medicine, inert dummies or decoys used to please the patient. As pest, placebo is annoyance, nuisance, noise, bias, or general non-specific effects to control in experiments so that researchers can demonstrate what's really happening. A third conception is of placebo as powerful mind-body medicine to be exploited itself. A fourth conception is "the history of the human need to swallow something" for its soothing effects (Bakal 1999). These conceptions are not the only choices and clearly they are mutually inconsistent. Placebo cannot be at the same time fake and real, or inert and powerful, if these opposites are to make sense, and similar contradictions appear in many other terms that have been used to express the notion of placebo.

Despite the importance and ubiquity of placebo in medicine, however, scientific investigation of what has come to be widely known as the placebo effect began only in the mid-twentieth century. Placebo and the placebo effect in the current incarnation are essentially post-World War II constructs. In 1945 the first medical paper with the word placebo in the title was published, at a time when it was not common to talk in terms of placebo effects (Shapiro and Shapiro 1997).

The leading view of placebo was shaped by Henry Beecher's (1955) frequently cited article in which he claimed that placebos have a powerful effect in precisely 35.2% ± 2.2% of cases in a variety of conditions. In a pioneering meta-analysis of previous research, Beecher reviewed 15 studies involving more than 1000 patients suffering from a range of conditions including severe wound pain, headache and nausea. The consistency of his observations led Beecher to believe that there was a common placebo mechanism in these cases deserving of further study. Since then general medical knowledge includes the notion that the placebo effect is about a third of the effect of any medical treatment. Or is it that a third of patients are placebo responders? Or is it a third of medical conditions that have placebo responders? Or a third of the good done by medicine? Or all of these thirds? Or is there any placebo effect at all? What Beecher's study showed is one of the common sources of confusion that suggests the need for closer examination of placebo.

From minority to majority

I am certainly not the first to call for change in terminology and for medicine to abandon current conceptions of placebo and placebo effects. Each generation reconsiders placebo in its own way, with rising and falling attention to associated medical mysteries, and researchers at various times and places have been predicting the demise of all things placebo. But while a small minority has called for change, the majority still accepts the concept of placebo and so will go to great lengths to interpret medicine in terms of placebo and often to stretch it to the breaking point to cover new observations and hypotheses. It's time now to respond to these calls for change by abandoning efforts to save the inherently flawed placebo concept.

The notion of placebo should be left to medical history. In the twentieth century, for instance, anthropologist Howard Stein (1983) wrote, "It is likely that the now-imaginary entity 'placebo' will suffer the same fate as did 'phlogiston' at the hands of Lavoisier and 'ether' at the hands of Einstein: it will become superfluous in the face of a more plausible model." But it apparently hasn't become superfluous yet and we're well into a shiny new century driving the same rusty old placebo model. Daniel Moerman (2002), also an anthropologist, has argued for abandoning the term placebo effect although not without exception: "I will argue that this is an unfortunate term, used carelessly for such a broad range of phenomena that we should probably abandon it; or, if we must keep it, we should only refer to the changes observed in the subjects in a control group in an experiment." I think we must not keep it at all.

Stein's mention of phlogiston refers to the early days of chemistry, before the discovery of the element oxygen, when a substance named phlogiston was proposed to explain what happens when something burns. Nobody knew exactly how phlogiston worked but that didn't stop its supporters from using the term as if phlogiston actually existed in the world. Eventually the notion of phlogiston was abandoned. Similarly, placebo was proposed to explain cures from substances and procedures without known medicinal powers. Both phlogiston and placebo were useful placeholders waiting for something better. Both were artifacts of particular viewpoints. The sooner the placebo habit follows phlogiston to the terminological graveyard, the better.

More recently, medical researcher Peter Gøtzsche (2007) writes, "We will need to accept that it has not been demonstrated convincingly that a placebo intervention can have an effect on the course of the disease... The technical term, a placebo effect, which cannot even be defined in a consistent way, should therefore be abandoned." That and other similar commentaries, however, have so far failed to dislodge placebo from its prominent place in medicine.

This is not to say there has been no movement at all toward something more sensible than placebo talk in medicine. Among theoreticians concerned with medical terminology, if not among medical practitioners, there has been a shift away from talking about placebo and placebo effects toward use of terms such as context and meaning. If this shift were to take hold in medicine generally, we would end up using words such as context effect or meaning response instead of placebo effect. But I want to go beyond adjusting the definition of placebo and placebo effects or offering alternative language for a concept that remains similar to placebo. I say placebo is an unnecessary construct that we would do better without altogether. We should expunge placebo and placebo effects from medical theory, research, training and practice.

What then? Since we tend to see what we look for, in future when we look, we will no longer see anything placebic in medicine. If we look at medicine differently we will see different things that will open up new possibilities. I outline some of those possibilities in the following chapters.

Aim of this discussion

I do not aim to solve all problems swirling around placebo and placebo effects in this discussion. The topic is too complex for that. Nor do I aim to substitute a few simple expressions to replace existing placebo language. In the past half-century, associated with the rise of clinical trial methodology in the 1950s, many people have contributed to the current conception of placebo. In the next half-century, I hope that many more people will at least ask whether they should continue puzzling over placebo or try a different approach like the one discussed here. Compared to their collective thoughts, I make only tentative proposals for what might emerge after placebo in medical theory, clinical practice, randomized controlled trials, bioethics, laws, regulations and other areas now conceived in terms of placebo.

I aim to show why we should abandon placebo now and how we might conceive of medicine after placebo. But I am not saying that eliminating a word here and there will by itself resolve or reduce the complexity of medicine. On the contrary, using the catch-all word placebo masks the complexity that needs to be examined. By the end of this discussion, I will have achieved my purpose if you have less confidence in the notion of placebo and more confidence in medicine after placebo. Or if you are at least persuaded that placebo must be considered from more than one viewpoint and that there is no single viewpoint that can ever make sense of placebo.

Viewpoints matter in medicine as they do in most endeavors. Mine is not just the familiar call for more research and funding, found at the end of many academic journal articles, but a call for different interpretations of what the research shows and will show. I also want to persuade you that different viewpoints are not only possible in medicine but are necessary. There is not one medical view from nowhere or everywhere, but multiple views of patients, physicians, theoreticians and many other variations. Patients see things from their experience that includes symptoms, worries, expectations and their own medical situations within their overall life contexts. Medical providers see things from different viewpoints based on their knowledge of the patient and their own backgrounds, training, specialties, roles and abilities. Researchers, politicians, pharmaceutical manufacturers and others interested in placebo have their own viewpoints.

Viewpoints also change over time. A viewpoint that is understood today in a particular way may not have been possible yesterday and may be unrecognizable tomorrow. Viewpoints are not only individual but may span organizations and societies. Points of view include not only scientistic biomedicine as practiced in the richest nations but also widely-held alternative views including traditional Chinese medicine, Ayurvedic medicine and a multitude of less widespread practices, and many do not currently view medicine in terms of placebo. It is impossible to address more than a fraction of existing viewpoints in this work despite their potential contribution to an examination of the notion of placebo. Considering more viewpoints after placebo will be a future project.

After placebo

The title *After Placebo* describes three aspects of this project with widespread implications for medical research and clinical practice:

Time: *After* refers to the future of medicine after it abandons the language of placebo. The phenomena that we associate with placebo today will not merely be given upgraded labels but will not be viewed as such in a post-placebo world.

Target: *After* also refers to searching after something; this work demonstrates the futility of sending a search party after the mythical placebo. That nobody has yet been able to define or delimit placebo, placebo effect or placebo responder suggests the illusory nature of their inquiry.

Temptation: *After* connotes the benefit expected after using a placebo treatment, the desire for a safe and plentiful magical cure-all. Can a placebo, or anything else, promise to make this dream come true?

The lone word *Placebo*, rather than *The Placebo*, in the title and throughout this discussion, also emphasizes the idea that placebo is not an ordinary article in the world but an imagined conceptual construct, so we should be mindful not to conceive of placebo as the thing, the placebo, the fake pill or the water injection, but instead to focus on placebo as a concept, just placebo, *tout court*. Or put in more formal terms, *placebo* is considered in this discussion to be a class of things while *the placebo* or *a placebo* is deemed to refer to a particular thing, an instance or member of the conceptual placebo class.

Conceptual habit

Given the notion of placebo, the usual habit is to try to explain it rather than challenge its foundations, to assume there is an existing thing in the world that placebo or some replacement word merely gives a name, without questioning that fundamental assumption. Placebo effects, for instance, may be reduced to brain effects or some other purported explanations. I do not look for an explanation of the ultimate, true, real placebo in terms of body parts, such as neurons and neurochemicals, or in changes visible during brain imaging. Nor do I look for a new and improved placebo concept that ingests these parts and grows into a more nuanced but wartier and hairier creature.

Many ideas in medicine, with names such as humors, bad air and vital or evil spirits, were considered useful for centuries but are now seen as less useful and indeed often harmful. Medicine formerly had labels for melancholics, morons, imbeciles, idiots and the lovesick. All of these terms in their day were believed to describe real observable medical phenomena. Witchcraft is another example. Witchcraft is no longer a notion accepted in current biomedicine, although related elements appear in reference to spiritual healing, medical superstition and voodoo death. Historian Stuart Clark (1997) begins his eight-hundred page history of witchcraft with this advice: "To make any kind of sense of the witchcraft beliefs of the past we need to begin with language." We must also begin with language when trying to make sense of present and past beliefs about placebo.

Old habits, including language habits, die hard and while we're constantly swimming in language, it's hard to notice when and which parts have become habitual. Some habits are not terribly misleading: we still refer to the horsepower of automobiles long after the horseless carriage chased most horse power from the streets. In casual everyday language, such old terms, including placebo, may have their place. People are still described as feeling sanguine, without any thought of the blood from which the word originates, or are said to be in good humor, without any commitment to ancient humoral theories of medicine. But when talking more rigorously, particularly in a current medical context, when understanding what works in medicine matters to suffering patients, in an age when medicine purports to be rational and scientific, old amorphous notions, including that of placebo, are not helpful and may be harmful.

Placebo has become a conceptual habit, as familiar and comfortable as an old shoe. Believers in the current placebo paradigm approach placebo as a normal, solvable, scientific puzzle that in time will become more like a squeaky new shoe. They suggest that understanding of placebo effects will eventually be found in the brain and solutions to placebo puzzles will be revealed by the methods of experimental science (for instance Benedetti 2009, Zubieta and Stohler 2009, Bingel 2011). To preserve the placebo notion, despite the many conceptual problems with placebo, they suggest tweaking it by, for example, extending placebo effects to include observations called placebo-related effects that appear in the absence of placebos (Benedetti 2008). Or they call for various alternative language that essentially replaces the word placebo with another term (for instance Brody 1980 and Moerman 2003 offer conceptions that advocate uses of the term meaning). There is even an attempt to explain changes in placebo observations over time in terms of the effects of human intention on physical matter, suggesting that the fundamental physics of our universe changed in the last three decades (Manek and Tiller 2011). An approach that rehabilitates, renames, extends or adjusts the placebo concept is more conservative and comfortable than abandoning it, even if that approach requires changing the physical universe to preserve placebo, as the ancients adjusted their physical universe to keep the Earth in its then preferred but ultimately untenable central place in the solar system.

Given that there could be such a category as placebo, to find confirming instances of placebo phenomena is not difficult. But whether placebo is replaced by a new term or stretched to include more of the conceptual landscape, neither approach moves us far beyond a world of mysterious placebo or placebo-related things. I take the more radical approach of eliminating the placebo category from our thinking. Then we stop saying placebo.

No simple answer

During the years in which I have been thinking about placebo, I have frequently asked people what they think a placebo is and what makes it work. Curiously, whether they are medical professionals or not, they almost always have a simple answer for a complex notion. For example, a family practitioner recently replied without hesitation, "It's just the power of suggestion." Things became less clear and more hesitant when I asked what is the power of suggestion and what makes that work.

The placebo effect is often taken as the answer in itself, not the question. How can a sugar pill relieve a headache? The answer might be, "Oh, that's the placebo effect." Or as one authority puts it, the answer is in "the efficacy of the placebo effect" (Taylor

1989). As if the word placebo itself contains a magical ingredient that makes us feel that we understand what's going on. As if placebo explains something, when it merely attaches a label to a thing, the sugar pill, and an observed effect, improvement in a patient, but fails to show how the fake pill is connected to the effect and explains nothing about why fake treatment appears to work sometimes in some people but not at other times or in other people.

Answers to questions about placebo eventually lead to unsatisfying clarifications and qualifications. For instance, to the question, "Can you give me an example of the placebo effect?" a common answer is something like, "when you give someone a pill with nothing in it but, say, sugar, and they get better." Follow that question with, "How can a sugar pill help someone get better?" Then the answers are more varied and more difficult. Ask, "What is the difference between the sugar put in a cup of coffee and a placebo sugar pill given to a patient?" The answer might be, "Well, everyone knows that the sugar pill is not a placebo until it is prescribed as a drug." If so, then at what point is the sugar transformed into a placebo? "The sugar all by itself is not the placebo." Alright, then what is the placebo? "The sugar pill together with the therapeutic context." Now we're plunging down into the placebo rabbit hole of context and leaving the simple answer far behind at the surface above.

Probe a bit more, and ask what exactly is the placebo effect. We will see throughout the following discussion that there is also no clear answer to that question. Merely because a patient improves after receiving a treatment, whether placebo or otherwise, does not demonstrate that the treatment makes any difference. The outcome might have been the same without the treatment. When the patient improves after swallowing a sugar pill, possible explanations for the improvement other than the biochemical nature of sugar include:

—wrong diagnosis: there was no disease
—placebo credited for other factors forgotten or ignored

—reported symptoms improved leaving the disease unchanged
—spontaneous recovery despite treatment
—the condition was self-limiting
—a chronic fluctuating condition happened to improve
—patient reported improvement to please the provider
—optimistic report of patient, provider or both

These are not the only explanations but they illustrate the confounding uncertainties in medicine that muddy any simple answer to questions about placebo or any clear statement of what placebo explains.

2 Placebo Language Matters

Until now in this discussion I have avoided the persistent problem of saying exactly what placebo is. As others have before me, I say there's no reasonable way to do so, but let's try.

In everyday conversation, a placebo is a particular kind of medical therapy, a dummy pill or procedure that resembles treatment. Typically, the pill contains a substance deemed to be medically inert, such as sugar or bread. The decoy is described by its provider as medically effective. Somehow, mysteriously, it appears to be effective in the patient.

Instead of a pill, the treatment could be practically anything, perhaps a water injection, perhaps rituals or words. An entertaining example that combines both a thing and a ritual is that of the physician who carried a large white tablet of vitamin C in tweezers, that implied the treatment was too powerful for bare hands. Dropped in a glass of water, magically the fizzling tablet relieved the patient's pain as no previous treatment had (Grünbaum 1985).

Fake surgery is another part of the placebo puzzle. If patients believe they have had surgery when they have only had the skin cut and sewn up again to fool them into thinking they have had surgery, that slice through the skin may apparently be as effective as the actual surgical procedure (Moseley et al. 2002). The bigger the fake pill, or the more invasive the procedure, the more effective it seems to be: painful fake injections and surgery seem to work better than less impressive fake interventions (Ernst 2001). There are countless other examples of the strangeness of placebo.

Various formal definitions of placebo, some resembling mathematical theorems and others with intricate clauses and subclauses resembling legal documents, have been proposed and hotly debated. For instance Shapiro and Shapiro (1997) devote a whole chapter to placebo semantics in their history called *The Powerful Placebo* in which they canvas many placebo definitions throughout history. They also contribute their own definition:

—A placebo is any therapy (or that component of any therapy) that is intentionally or knowingly used for its nonspecific, psychological, or psychophysiological, therapeutic effect, or that is used for a presumed specific therapeutic effect on a patient, symptom, or illness but is without specific activity for the condition being treated.

—A placebo, when used as a control in experimental studies, is a substance or procedure that is without specific activity for the condition being treated.

—The placebo effect is the nonspecific psychological or psychophysiological therapeutic effect produced by a placebo.

Immediately following this layered collage the Shapiros add, "In other words …" and continue to clarify their proposal with even more nuances than in the definition itself. Earlier, Grünbaum (1985) and Brody (1985) also provided lengthy examples of conjectured and refuted definitions of placebo and placebo effect. More recently, Harrington (2006) offers not one but three choices from placebo history: an inert substance that looks like real medicine, or the non-specific effect that must be controlled in clinical trials, or a powerful mind-body phenomenon for use in medicine.

By contrast, Gøtzsche (1994) declared, "I have tried to define placebo in an unambiguous, logically consistent, and testable way, and I have failed." He suggested taking a pragmatic view; a decade later in one of their systematic reviews, Hróbjartsson and Gøtzsche (2004) avoided the definition problem by letting the word mean whatever the author chooses: "We pragmatically defined a placebo intervention as any intervention, which was clearly labeled a placebo in a trial report."

Neuroscientist Fabrizio Benedetti (2009) attempts a succinct definition: "To give a placebo to a group of patients means to give a sham medical treatment. Accordingly, the therapeutic outcome is called 'placebo effect', which means the effect that follows administration of the placebo." This definition comes shortly after an explanation of sham treatment in history that concludes by saying that placebo is the more recent word for sham treatment. So "sham mesmerism" and "sham homeopathy" is replaced today by "placebo mesmerism" and "placebo homeopathy."

If sham and placebo are synonyms, however, then the circular definition says only that placebo is placebo: substituting placebo for sham in Benedetti's definition we get "To give a placebo to a group of patients means to give a placebo medical treatment." Placebo cannot add much to the conversation as a direct replacement for sham. Indeed sham is more of a description, not the whole thing in itself, only a property that connotes deception among other properties attributed to placebo. Note also that the definition refers to a group, so it addresses groups in clinical trials and not individual patients in clinical practice or elsewhere.

The latter part of the definition is another circular reference: "Accordingly, the therapeutic outcome is called 'placebo effect', which means the effect that follows the administration of the placebo." Again placebo effect is defined in relation to placebo which is recursively defined in terms of its effect. Benedetti notes that these definitions have caused confusion, although he refers only to other explanatory factors such as spontaneous remission or expectation of therapeutic benefit. But the confusion is conceptual not just empirical. Patients may be seen to improve and the improvement may be explained as spontaneous or in some other terms, but confusion about what placebo is and how we can know what it does remains in these deceptively self-referent definitions.

Definitional problems are not definitive, only suggestive. Definitions are not always possible or helpful. Not only placebos but vast ranges of things elude definition. This is not the eternal problem of defining abstract terms like truth, justice or art, however. Nor is the definitional problem for placebo merely a matter of vagueness or generality. Placebo refers to a class of things that researchers and clinicians say they administer to patients. Placebo has been viewed in medicine as a particular observable thing, yet a thing that defies definition. The perennial failure to define placebo in complete or consistent terms constrains theorizing about the undefined object of any placebo theory.

Will you be understood if you say placebo effect?

Among many reasons to stop talking in terms of placebo, consider whether you will be understood when you say placebo effect or, according to recent fashion, when you pluralize them as placebo effects. Harrington (2011) writes optimistically that, "We all have a certain understanding of what is meant by the placebo effect: the tendency of patients to report feeling better or otherwise having a response to a drug or treatment that is known or later discovered to be inert or ineffective." Yet can we all have a certain understanding when placebo effects have been constructed in many forms, not all mutually compatible?

Often a distinction is drawn between the desired therapeutic placebo effect to be encouraged in clinical practice and the nuisance placebo effect to be controlled or eliminated in a clinical trial. Consider for instance a distinction offered by a clinical trialist who explained that the placebo effect is when you specifically tell someone that the sugar pill will stop their pain. In his view that is different from the situation in blind randomized clinical trials where typically one does not even have to talk or think much about a placebo effect when designing a trial. Given the predicted outcome in the control group, the appropriate trial size can be calculated to show a difference between treatment groups. After all, the placebo control for a typical trial, whether in pill, capsule or some other visible form, is made to be indistinguishable from the experimental treatment so everybody thinks the treatments are the same. The implication of similar widely held views is that there is a baseline psychological effect in clinical trials that can be routinely subtracted from every participant's results to reveal the difference between treatments.

Just as it's convenient to divide treatments into exclusive opposites such as specific or non-specific, effective or ineffective, active or inert, it's also convenient to divide effects between clinical practice and experimental trials. Given those alternative boxes, arguments can be made for bifurcating all observations and neatly categorizing them accordingly.

More options are available than the simple, yet deceptive, division between any of these alternatives. Listeners could hear you speaking of a wide variety of things when you say placebo effect, including the following non-exhaustive possibilities:

—effects of fake treatment
—effects of patient-provider interaction
—effects of the specific act of treatment

—effects of the general context of treatment

—effects of a sub- (or non-) therapeutic dose (not a fake)

—effects of mind (or brain) on body

—effects of expectation and hope

—effects constructed by biomedical observers

—general metaphor for deception (as in mere placebo)

—improvement in the placebo control group of an experiment

—improvement in the placebo control group minus other factors such as spontaneous improvement

—non-specific effects of treatment (an issue of specificity)

—non-characteristic effects of treatment (an issue of deemed characteristics)

—responses of neurotic personalities with imagined or feigned conditions

—responses of particularly suggestible and optimistic personalities (responders?) with observable (objective?) conditions

—common effects of all medical treatments throughout all of medical history

It's not clear which observations fit into which of these overlapping descriptions. If we are all to have a certain understanding of what is meant by placebo effect, a greater certainty is needed in medicine than in everyday conversation. But there is no greater certainty in medicine when it comes to anything about placebo. Surveys show that physicians and patients vary widely in their understanding and explanation of placebo effects and mind-body medicine (Sherman and Hickner 2007, Chen and Johnson 2009, Clifford 2011). Unless you have the time and energy to be extremely specific about what you mean, you take your chances with at least these possibilities, among others.

If the notion of placebo effect is not the main focus of discussion, the chances of negotiating common understanding become smaller. Fleck (1979) describes a vivid example of medical historians debating whether a modern diagnosis can be made from an ancient medical text. In support of the possibility, one speaker claims that diseases remain unchanged, but that claim was not specifically taken up in the conversation. So a notion of unchanging disease became an axiom in the debate although very likely none of the speakers accepted the claim that diseases remain unchanged— "Very often it is impossible to find any originator for an idea generated during discussion and critique. Its meaning changes repeatedly; it is adapted and becomes common property. Accordingly it achieves a superindividual value, and becomes an axiom, a guideline for thinking." Similarly talk of the placebo effect or placebo effects becomes axiomatic, despite at least a dozen interpretations that no debater can support all at once.

In the interest of brevity, let's consider only a few of the many possible confusions when you say placebo effect. Will you be understood to mean the effects of a fake drug or procedure, or will your listener also envision the effects of a limited or unconventional use of a genuine drug? Do placebo effects mean the improvement in the control group or some part of the improvement or some part of the group? Have you distinguished the effects of concealed treatments meant to fool patients in clinical practice from the effects of control treatments given to informed consenting groups of experimental subjects? Do you include all kinds of mind-body interaction or something limited to patient-provider contexts? Is the type of mind-body interaction that is called the placebo effect the same as the psychological or psychophysiological effect? Is expectation included in the notion of patient-provider context or is expectation something else? Where do conditioning and learning fit in this picture? Are superstitious associations included in placebo conditioning? Are those who respond to sugar pills as adults also those whose caregivers conditioned them as children with candy or a spoonful of sugar to soothe their distress? Are placebo effects greater in a special kind of responsive person? Can you explain how the majority of patients, the placebo non-responders, apparently fail to show effects of learning, conditioning and expectation in a medical context?

If there is any law-like causal relationship, it is the notional one that associates placebo with those effects that don't fit more conveniently elsewhere in biomedicine. A placebo seems to produce an effect when we don't understand the cause. If we do have a causal explanation, the language changes: we don't call it a placebo. Everyone says placebo effects while few say placebo causes. The entity called placebo seems inseparable from knowledge of that entity's effects. The term placebo effect then suggests a simple causal model, a one-to-one relation:

A placebo causes the placebo effect.

The indefinite article, a placebo or any placebo, or indeed anything, resolves down to the definite article for the placebo effect, the effect of improvement for any condition after any placebo treatment. If a placebo is viewed as a fake treatment, such as a sugar pill or water injection represented to the patient as something else, then the relation is:

A fake treatment causes the placebo effect.

Behind this apparent simplicity lie many complexities. Although pills and needles are real things that can be observed in the world, it's not at all clear that placebos are real. The apparently real things involved in placebo effects are difficult to pin down with any precision. In the absence of a person in a medical context, the thing itself is just a lump of sugar or a squirt of water. Pills and fluid-filled syringes are visible things, but it's not the sugar or the pill, not the static visible thing, that attracts the name placebo. To say placebo is to invoke a complex, multi-level, self-referent network of beliefs, expectations, events, dynamics, mechanisms, observations, people, processes and more that are associated with puzzling effects correlated with medical treatments.

Also complex are the contentious concepts of medicine, disease, illness and health that underlie the notion of placebo. The dominant methodology in biomedicine for demonstrating what cures disease and what relieves suffering, the randomized placebo-controlled clinical trial, is an exercise in observing correlations when different groups receive different treatments, not an exercise in devising models of causal mechanisms in clinical practice. All of which is to suggest that the misleading simple model:

A placebo causes the placebo effect.

hides too many issues to be useful. The model is only marginally improved by pluralizing, as in:

Placebos cause placebo effects.

This move is advocated by Fabrizio Benedetti whose book *Placebo Effects: understanding the mechanisms in health and disease* (2009) is a reference text for the current biomedical view of placebo effects. He chose the plural *Effects* in the title to emphasize that there isn't just one placebo effect but many. Benedetti would also extend the term placebo effects beyond placebo to include what he calls placebo-related effects that occur in the absence of placebos. In this conception,

Non-placebos may cause placebo-related effects.

His main project has been to elucidate the brain mechanisms associated with placebo effects. Although he does not explicitly say that mechanisms are causal explanations, that appears to be the case. He writes, "The placebo effect is a real psychobiological phenomenon whereby the brain is actively involved and anticipates a clinical benefit. Therefore, this book strives to make it clear that when we study the placebo, we are actually studying how the brain anticipates an event in the clinical setting." That description raises many difficult questions including the following:

—What is observable in relation to placebo?

Placebo is usually described in terms of placebo effect, as in the above examples. In the current paradigm, almost anything can have a placebo effect (Shapiro and Shapiro 1997, Bausell 2007). If placebo is a general property of almost anything, how is it that the property is only observable as an effect? Placebo is not a property like weight or size. Is placebo conceived as an invisible force, like magnetism, that becomes observable through its effects? Yet nobody speaks of placebo forces, only placebo effects.

—How is brain related to mind?

Neuroscientists often refer to the brain actively doing things, such as anticipating, that others have attributed to the mind or person. Talk of brains thinking, expecting, anticipating and so on appears to avoid persistent disputes about relations between mind and body, the mind-body dualism that has bothered so many others. Since it does not mention the mind, the description therefore appears to avoid any metaphysical mind-body separation. To address the problem of dualism built into our language, the solution appears to be disturbingly simple: just say brain instead of mind, since we all know that the brain is part of the body, and we can therefore look for answers in observable body parts or in a chimerical brain-body.

So earlier in this discussion, instead of saying that many people have contributed to the received notion of placebo, I could have said that many brains have contributed. Or many brain-bodies. Or bodies with brains. Instead of trying to change your mind about how you think of placebo, I could have exhorted you to change your brain. No need to worry then about how the mind or consciousness or thought can appear among biochemicals and cells and perhaps some day in computer chips. It's all in the brain; in this conception, mind and brain are the same thing seen from different viewpoints and described by different language.

But replacing mind with brain does not actually resolve these problems. It merely replaces mind-body dualism with brain-body dualism. Nowhere in the neuro-description is a person *who* anticipates, rather than the brain or mind *that* anticipates. The person's feelings, thoughts and mind, conscious and unconscious, function not just within the brain or brain-body but in the person's whole environment within and around the person's brain-body. Context appears to be central to explanations of placebo, and it is the person, not just the brain, that has the context in which to do things such as anticipate.

—What is "psychobiological"?

Is psychobiological the same as, or reducible to, neurobiological? Benedetti (2009) refers on the same page both to "real psychobiological phenomenon" and to "real neurobiological placebo response" and then there are references to the study of placebo as the study of psychosocial context then as alternately psychosocial or psychological component. How is a component, that is, a part of a person, related to the person in context, that is, a whole person? Neuro-things are in the realm of the brain while psycho-things are in the realm of the mind-brain, all of which are in a person, and socio-things involve more than one person. How are these things related to each other? Placebo in a neuro-conception is in the brain that anticipates, yet at the same time spans every realm from the neuro- to the bio- to the psycho- and even the socio- realms as both part and whole.

The terms psychobiological, psychosocial, social and psychological, which do not refer only to mechanisms, are mixed with the main focus, neurobiological mechanisms. Problems arise when generalizing across so many concepts and levels of organization. For instance, in the case of alcohol abuse, "there is only modest evidence to support powerful placebo effects across different domains of social behaviour" (Benedetti 2009). Generalizations crossing different domains are conceptual, not just matters of evidence from more research.

—What is "real" or "true" in relation to placebo?

This question focuses on the desire to find the real or true placebo as in "real psychobiological phenomenon" or "true psychobiological placebo effect." The idea is to distinguish placebo effects, real and true, from spontaneous improvement, bias and other explanations for the observed effects of treatment. Such a positivist biomedical view, in which there is an objective, impersonal reality corresponding to the claimed truth and reality of placebo, merits examination, particularly given the role of belief, expectation, context and other subjective, personal aspects associated with placebo.

—What is the connection between clinical context and placebo research?

The definition above refers to clinical benefit and clinical context. Much placebo research takes place outside the everyday clinic in controlled experiments. The applicability of this extra-clinical work to the clinic cannot be assumed and merits examination, particularly in light of claims that vast regions of the medical landscape, including most forms of complementary and alternative medicine, are essentially placebo.

Placebos as commonly misconceived

Common misconceptions about placebo are many, including: a placebo is an inert substance, about a third of people respond to placebos, only neurotic personalities respond to placebos, placebos relieve only pain and anxiety, placebo effects are not long-lasting and placebos are harmless. These and many other misconceptions have been frequently raised in the literature. Wall (1996), for instance, catalogs six placebo myths:

1. the placebo differentiates between organic and mental disease
2. the placebo is the equivalent of no therapy
3. a fixed fraction of patients respond to placebos
4. placebo responders have a special mentality
5. pain is a multidimensional experience and the placebo affects only a part
6. the placebo effect may be dissected to reveal the pure therapeutic action

Persistent myths and misconceptions such as these among health professionals raise central questions about the nature of placebo. For the purposes of this discussion, they also raise questions about whether the best way forward is to mount heroic efforts to slay each myth and reverse each misconception, to cite study after study in support of a particular conception of placebo and debate the merits of each conception, or to stop saying placebo and bury the myths and misconceptions together with placebo terminology.

3 Mr Wright's Case

A famous example illustrating many placebo matters is the case of a patient named Mr Wright that has been frequently cited as one of the most dramatic validations of placebo. His case was so important to medical historian Anne Harrington (2008) that she begins the first chapter of her book on the history of mind-body medicine with the words, "Mr Wright was a very sick man." Philosopher Dylan Evans (2003) describes the story of Mr Wright as the, "one case recorded in the medical literature that looks like a case of the placebo response curing cancer." Harrington uses the Wright case to introduce the historical narrative she calls the power of suggestion while Evans concludes that the most likely explanation for Wright's dramatic improvement and decline was coincidence.

Projective hearsay

Curiously, everybody who mentions Mr Wright can only quote someone who quotes someone else. For what we know of Mr Wright's medical history is only weak hearsay evidence of the kind often associated with miracles that happened long ago, to someone else, somewhere else, and so cannot be directly verified. Despite his prominence in the placebo literature, his story essentially rests on 15 short paragraphs of indirect evidence reported more than a half-century ago. Moreover, those paragraphs are not directly from his oncologist or anyone at all who examined him but are from psychologist Bruno Klopfer who got the story by personal communication from one of Mr Wright's physicians. Klopfer's (1957) paper cited by everyone who discusses Mr Wright was not even a formal scientific report about Mr Wright's case but rather was Klopfer's presidential address for the annual meeting of the Society of Projective Techniques.

Klopfer explains that Mr Wright had lymphosarcoma with, among other observations, "Huge tumor masses, all the size of oranges... in the neck, axilla, groins, chest and abdomen." He was "febrile, gasping for air, completely bedridden" and was not expected to live more than two weeks. But he was apparently convinced that the new drug Krebiozen that was being tested at his physician's clinic would save him. Krebiozen was later shown to be a fraudulent treatment, "containing a white powder said to come from the blood of horses injected with a microorganism responsible for 'lumpy jaw in cattle'" (Shapiro and Shapiro 1997).

Mr Wright received one injection on a Friday. By Monday he was walking around the ward and, "The tumor masses had melted like snow balls on a hot stove, and in only those few days, they were half their original size!" (Klopfer 1957). Within 10 days Mr Wright was discharged and flew home in his own plane.

Unfortunately Mr Wright heard discouraging news from clinical trials of Krebiozen and relapsed, "after two months of practically perfect health." So his physician deceived Mr Wright by saying that the relapse was because the drug deteriorates on standing, and he would now receive super-refined double-strength product. "With much fanfare and putting on quite an act," his physician administered an injection of fresh water and, "Recovery from his second near-terminal state was even more dramatic than the first: Tumor masses melted, chest fluid vanished, he became ambulatory, and even went back to flying again." But after another two months, Krebiozen was reported to be a worthless cancer treatment. "Within a few days of this report, Mr Wright was re-admitted to the hospital in extremis. His faith was now gone, his last hope vanished, and he succumbed in less than two days."

Mr Wright's story was one of 24 cases studied by Klopfer. His main interest was in Rorschach (inkblot) tests of cancer patients.

In particular, he wondered whether he could guess, from reading Rorschach test reports, which patients had slow-growing or fast-growing cancer. Klopfer claimed that he was able to guess correctly, not every time, but better than chance. In the presidential address he outlines his hypothesis, then at the end of his presentation he describes a case that fooled him, where the Rorschach reports indicated a slow-growing cancer but the patient had fast-growing cancer. That patient, Mr Wright, was never seen by Klopfer. Yet from its humble origin in hearsay evidence used to explain a psychologist's hypothesis about the prognostic power of inkblots, Mr Wright's case has grown to assume a remarkably strong following in the placebo literature. It is ironic that Klopfer dealt in Rorschach tests, since their questionable power has been linked to the power of the experimenter's suggestion, as have placebos (Masling 1997).

Questionable power

Does Mr Wright's case demonstrate the power of placebo? Of the mind over cancer? Consider alternative accounts. One possibility is that the reported observations were not accurate either as originally conveyed by his physician or as reported second-hand by Klopfer. For instance, the case as reported says Mr Wright received, "no other treatment outside of a single useless 'shot'." But he was in a hospital and earlier in the report we are told that milky fluid was drawn from his chest every other day and he was also receiving oxygen by mask frequently as well as sedatives. Are these not "other treatment"? That is, Klopfer focused on the drug, the magic bullet, as the only biomedical treatment to the exclusion of other activities that might also be considered treatment. Likely there were additional treatments omitted from the informal report.

There is also no way of knowing whether Mr Wright, like so many desperate and dying patients, tried all sorts of treatments in the hope of recovery, some of which he might not have discussed with his physicians. As an aircraft owner and pilot who flew home in his own plane, Mr Wright apparently had the means to pay for special treatments. The whole story framed as placebo drama disappears if it was merely an exaggeration incompletely or inaccurately reported.

Let us assume, however, for the purposes of this discussion, that the reported observations were complete and accurate. Another possibility is that the course of his disease may have been a series of roller-coaster ups and downs, with a cycle of around two months, unrelated to water injection and hopes for Krebiozen. Perhaps needless to say, correlation is not causation. Tumors may appear, disappear and reappear. His physicians may have interpreted outside influences such as Krebiozen, the injection of water, other interventions and Mr Wright's lack of faith from reading of the failure of Krebiozen, as the power behind the roller coaster. But perhaps the momentum of the disease would have carried or followed Mr Wright up and down in any event. Perhaps outsiders only believed they were pushing him up and down. Mr Wright's case was a classic anecdote. But as hard cases make bad law, single cases make dubious medical theory.

Expected base rate

An important but seldom-discussed aspect of dramatic exemplars such as Mr Wright's story is the expected base rate of spontaneous remissions and regressions for the disease that Mr Wright had. To declare that his case is unusual we need to know what is usual. What makes his case stand out from countless others is that it defies expectation or prediction. This man was not expected to survive.

His imminent death was predicted. His cancer was not expected to disappear spontaneously. Yet it seems to have disappeared at least twice.

Events that defy expectation depend on a base rate of occurrences for each prediction. We are not surprised when the sun appears at the horizon as predicted because it happens regularly every morning. Given the much less common and less predictable event of death by lightning strike, it's headline news when someone gets hit by lightning. It's even more newsworthy when someone survives a lightning strike, or by analogy, when Mr Wright, stricken with cancer, recovers twice.

At least three different predictions appear in Mr Wright's case: time until death, chance of regression, likelihood of relapse. All have different rates, ranges of predictability and margins of error. The body is constantly fending off disease, so any surprise at spontaneous recovery must come from more than the ordinary experience of getting better. Yet it is impossible to know how often the body successfully defends itself. Things in the body invisibly come and go and may not be investigated or reported.

In a review of regression cases in cancer, Papac (1996) states that most patients who regress ultimately relapse, just as Mr Wright did. Papac cites various case examples and notes the variable natural history of lymphoma that suggests regression in lymphoma cases may not be uncommon. In light of those observations, Mr Wright's case was to some extent expected, not a one-of-a-kind miracle. That he regressed twice, both times after receiving an injection, may appear to be a scientific confirmation, a brief clinical trial, of the power of faith in an injection and therefore of placebo. But two heads in a row do not demonstrate anything about the possible bias of a flipped coin. Or if this case is conceived in terms of low-probability events, such as the uncommon spontaneous remission of cancer, then in a similar vein, a couple of lottery wins by the same person sooner or later are inevitable at some time in history somewhere in the world, and do not demonstrate a lottery effect or any other mysterious lottery mechanism or unusual causal story. The indicia of placebo science cannot be firmly attached to Mr Wright's case.

Mr Wright's case is also similar to another dramatic example of regression made famous in the controversial quest by Nobel laureate Linus Pauling and Ewan Cameron to validate vitamin C treatment for cancer. The case was succinctly described as follows:

> In 1975, we reported the remarkable case of a 42-year-old man with histologically proven widely disseminated reticulum cell sarcoma who, in a remarkably short time, appeared to enjoy not one, but two, complete spontaneous regressions of his fatal illness. Both these regressions coincided exactly in time with intravenous high-dose ascorbate administration, and it seemed reasonable to conclude that this unconventional therapy must have been responsible for his excellent responses (Campbell et al. 1991).

It is instructive that the authors say the regressions coincided with therapy. Then they make the tenuous leap to a causal story of therapy being responsible and claim that such a conclusion seemed reasonable. How insidiously and smoothly a slim correlation morphs into a strong causation. Was it the vitamin C or the placebo effect of the treatment that was responsible for the excellent responses? Placebo proponents might prefer the latter explanation in this case as in Mr Wright's case. Vitamin proponents might prefer the former. In medicine after placebo, however, neither explanation seems reasonable.

Not knowing

With that background, can we conclude that Mr Wright is the world's best example of a placebo responder or not? It's difficult to say anything conclusive when confronted with a story of the form "there was this one guy who..." (Hunter 1986). If we say Krebiozen and the water injection did the work, or include Mr Wright's beliefs and the fanfare provided by his physicians, the answer is still yes or no. Perhaps Krebiozen and water injection had something to do with his trajectory in this case. Perhaps not. Observations don't explain themselves in any event, so we have to choose among competing theories. Is placebo the best explanation? Or is it coincidence? Bias? Error? Fiction? We just don't know enough to explain the apparent correlation between interventions and his condition.

Not knowing and not being able to explain may be uncomfortable. But we should resist the urge to accept a convenient placebic explanation that only relieves our intellectual discomfort with our own ignorance. Admitting lack of knowledge is better than plastering over problems by saying placebo. There is no need to divide the world into real effects and placebo effects. But if that's what you do, then you'll probably observe placebo effects in Mr Wright, just as those ancients, whose humoral medicine had exactly four humors, observed all four of them, not three and a third, not sixty-two.

In the placebo literature, Mr Wright's case may have reached the popular viral stage where it appears to be brought to our attention in part because it is available in memory after having so often been brought to our attention. For instance, while explaining the placebo effect, psychologist Shelley Taylor (1989) quotes the description of Mr Wright's case by the popular mind-body medicine advocate Bernie Siegel. She warns against overgeneralizing: "The dilemma with the individual case is that one can never conclusively demonstrate that a particular factor, such as an illusion, led to a particular error or problem. One also cannot judge the adequacy of a process solely on the basis of its outcome." In spite of her own warning, the received notion of placebo effect is such an insidious fixture that this expert, in a book devoted to positive illusions and self-deception, cites Mr Wright's apparent positive example of placebo-induced cancer regression but does not weigh it against the many and more common failures of placebo treatment for cancer.

We will return for a brief placebo-free account of Mr Wright's case but first we must consider the many shortcomings of placebo language and theory.

4 Placebo by Any Other Name

Practical people who just want to get their work done might ask if this is all just semantics. They find the placebo effect to be a useful notion and even if it's not perfect, they don't see much wrong with it. Anyway, what does it matter whether we call it the placebo effect or something else? A placebo by any other name would please as much.

We could continue to say that placebo and the placebo effect are what they are no matter what they are called, as for example Macedo et al. (2003) do: "one issue seems unquestionable: the placebo effect is present in clinical practice and in clinical trials, no matter which name we choose to call it." A similar laissez-faire attitude appears in Cherniak (2010): "However a placebo is defined, information about the placebo effect garnered from clinical trials, may suggest potential therapeutic uses." But to say "which name we choose to call it" is to presume there is an "it" that lurks out there in the world needing to be named, independent of language and the network of associations among words.

The word placebo imports a variety of assumptions about medicine and people. Placebo is not merely a name that describes something in the world but a model that constructs something that is not in the world. My view is that the label placebo cannot be attached meaningfully to any medical phenomena.

We no longer conceive of entities in the world associated with old names such as phlogiston, humors and vital spirits, just as we should no longer look for the "it" of placebo. As with phlogiston, for instance, which yielded to more plausible models and explanations for combustion, the absence of placebo notions will make way for new models and explanations in medicine.

Those who want to keep the notion of placebo might attack as being hypocritical what I have been saying in this discussion so far. They might say: you have been using the word placebo all along so obviously you can't stop saying placebo and we can't either! How can you argue against placebo while using terms dependent on placebo?

My response is that I have no choice but to start with the language of placebo. How could I refer to the concept of placebo effects without saying placebo effects? An awkward solution would be to always use quotation marks around "placebo" or I could say so-called placebo or some other qualifier to emphasize the questionable nature of placebo. To avoid such awkwardness, however, the solution used in this discussion is simply to assume that an appropriate qualifier is attached to each use of the word placebo until some future time when we refer to placebo only as an artifact of a previous era, just as we do not need to say to someone "You're in so-called good humor today" to show that we no longer believe in the four humors of ancient medicine.

My use of other terms such as fake treatment, which assumes that we can make a distinction between fake and real treatment, might also be criticized. Whether a treatment is fake or real is one of the very things that placebo is used to investigate. But we have to start somewhere.

The unusual nature of the word placebo in medicine is illustrated by frequent etymological reminders in medical literature, often accompanied by religious references, about the Latin origin of the word placebo. Something special is behind the frequent inclusion of parenthetical explanations attached to placebo, often in the form: (Latin for "I shall please") and to nocebo (Latin for "I harm"). These dusty historical explanations appear even in current medical literature that usually has no space or editorial patience for such unscientific digressions. Science and medicine borrow Latin words at every turn, but not many scientific or medical papers devote prized parts of their limited word quotas to discussing the Latin origins of the word calcium or phrases such as the temporal fenestrae of the cranium. Current research papers on malaria are unlikely to include reminders about medieval theories of bad air and their connection to old Italian language from which the word malaria came.

No doubt nocebo is a less familiar term for many people but for whom is the word placebo so unfamiliar that tracing it to back to liturgical Latin is necessary? Surely it is not less familiar to the average reader of medical literature than words like calcium or fenestrae, which are not usually accompanied in medical papers with parentheses such as calcium (Latin *calx, calcis,* lime) or fenestrae (Latin plural of *fenestra,* window). Is it because more concrete and comprehensible notions than placebo. such as calcium, bad air or window, do not typically need that parenthetical scholarly boost to their credibility? Placebo seems to demand a more descriptive, qualitative discourse than biomedicine typically prefers. Placebo language is different.

It's important not to reify placebo by explaining its Latin origin and thereby incorrectly assume that placebos and placebo effects are obvious things in the medical world that have been around for centuries and that everyone understands what the name means. Placebo does not only label a thing, a sugar pill or fake injection, but encapsulates contemporary ideas about humans and our beliefs, bodies and behavior.

Concepts and categories influence what we consider to be real and what we consider to be real, in turn, influences what we accept as concepts. Many others have discussed the importance of categorical constructs in our thinking (from ancient philosophers to recent examples such as Lakoff 1987 and Taleb 2007). Placebo, and its negative shadow nocebo, shape how we think. They are not neutral words, if indeed neutral words exist. They are Latinate, medical-sounding words with authority and a scent of disinfectant and other associations that cannot entirely be captured in words apart from experience. They support a particular world view, not limited to linguistic habits but extending to images, diagrams, models, feelings and imagination, a view that contains those named things. Or at least a subset of possible views that use placebo in various untranslatable, incommensurable ways. Placebo and nocebo are persuasive rhetorical devices, as terms such as *terrorists* brands enemies and *freedom-fighters* promotes allies, that may refer to the same individuals depending on who is talking. Placebo rhetoric extends to associated words too. Placebo detractors link placebo with diminutive words, as in mere placebo, while placebo supporters prefer more expansive associations such as powerful placebo and magic cure.

To say that placebo is something inert, yet powerful at the same time, requires a modifier: the word inert has to be modified to make sense of "inert and powerful" by adding terms such as "chemically inert." So placebo has been described as chemically inert but clinically powerful. The same modifier cannot be attached simultaneously to both terms, however, as for instance "chemically inert but chemically powerful at the same time", because that doesn't make sense. Placebo makes a mysterious bridge between "chemically" and "clinically" without explaining the link between the inert chemical and the non-specific clinical effects.

Scientific hypotheses, theories and observations cannot make a meaningless concept meaningful; more observations cannot make sense of inert things causing effects. Observations can provide a basis for causal inferences, but we must also have a sensible hypothesis. Naming something placebo determines how we hypothesize about it. Placebo is a word that may never be adequately grasped, but we cannot avoid choosing words instead of jumping directly into observations of placebo effects.

If your conception of the world includes something called a unicorn, then when you see a horse-like creature at sunrise partly hidden behind golden tree leaves, not just the word unicorn comes to mind but the possibility arises that what you see is not a mere horse. The language we use shapes our metaphysics and epistemology, our theories and observations. The unicorn called placebo has become too engrained in our thinking.

Engrained, entrenched placebo

Indeed, not only is placebo language engrained, but a review of placebo effects published in a leading medical journal, *The Lancet*, argues that placebo is so engrained in the literature that we can't do anything about it now:

> ...placebo terminology, despite its defects, is too engrained in the scientific literature to replace it at this time, especially in the absence of a satisfactory alternative (Finniss et al. 2010).

The engrained placebo metaphor accords with a similar reluctant acceptance of the entrenched placebo:

> Although the placebo concept is fraught with confusion, the terminology of the 'placebo effect' and the 'placebo response' is entrenched in the language of biomedicine and unlikely to be abandoned in the near future (Miller et al. 2009).

The authors do not speculate on why placebo talk has become so engrained or entrenched. It could be a result of confidence in our current knowledge, conventions, research programs and methodologies for generating future knowledge. It could be confirmation bias that has been said to be generally responsible for the persistence of outdated theories. It could be that placebo serves the interests of those who rely on the concept. The boundaryless scope of placebo permits every constituency to claim ownership and to use it in their own interests. Pharmaceutical manufacturers, for instance, benefit from the entrenched linear view of placebo that permits them unfettered choice of placebo controls that are used by comparison to distinguish their profitable products. It could be reluctance to take on such a daunting task as elimination of the engrained or entrenched placebo, among other possibilities. Any reconceptualization of placebo could cast into doubt past research programs and present careers. There does not appear to be a grand conspiracy to preserve the placebo concept in medicine. But as in any human endeavor, there is a weight of history that resists change. Medicine is a particularly conservative endeavor and the history of medicine has been a history of delay and resistance to change (Wootton 2006).

For whatever reasons, placebo terminology remains despite its acknowledged defects. I agree that the terminology should not be replaced. But I oppose waiting and searching for a satisfactory alternative. Rather, engrained entrenched placebo terminology should be excised wherever possible. Now not later. Eventually, as with any change in world view, we can stop trying to solve received scientific puzzles engendered by defective concepts. That placebo terminology is widely accepted by experts to be defective is reason enough to move beyond placebo although, or even because, we have become addicted to the familiar, if inscrutable, placebo habit of speaking.

To those practical people who say that placebo is a useful word, and they need a name for it, I say placebo is a misleading word and not a construct that we need. The transition to new language may take time during which both old and new conceptions will appear side by side. But eventually we should use placebo terminology less and less until it becomes a mere curiosity from the past.

The burden of placebo proof

A first-order burden of proof is whether an observation is or is not a placebo effect. This is the typical level addressed in reports of experiments such as placebo-controlled clinical trials. A second-order burden lies on theoreticians who say the category of placebo describes things in the world. The same could be said of those who disdain theory and merely say that placebo is a useful grouping of observed effects that need a name whether that name is placebo or some other name.

The burden of proof could be stated in terms of signal detection theory, which distinguishes four states when considering the truth of a detected signal: true, false, false positive or false negative. At a first-order level, deeming something to be a placebo effect, when it is not, would be a false positive.

Allan and Siegel (2002) go so far as to propose that placebo effects can be errors in observations made by patients. They say that observing placebo effects can be a form of false positive error in which a definite placebo signal is detected from ambiguous stimuli. When a patient is looking for a single cause in the haystack of causes in medicine, the words of an expert who declares where to find the cause are persuasive. When an expert suggests that an observation is a placebo effect, an ambiguous signal can be parsed as a certain placebo effect.

As signal detection theory applies to individual placebo observations, it could also apply to the notion of placebo at a second-order theoretical level. At a second-order level, deeming the category of placebo to be representative of the world, or perhaps merely useful, when it is not, would be a false positive. What supports the claim that the notion of placebo represents the world, or for the pragmatic empiricist, that the notion of placebo does any work? To the extent that there is uncertainty about the placebo category, we should not assume that placebo is an appropriate construct to wrap around things we see in the world. We should not take the relatively short scientific history of placebo, less than a century, as the enduring nature of things instead of the long history of medical concepts that have come and gone.

The likelihood that a scientific claim is reliable depends, among other things, on the probability of the claim prior to the research (Ioannidis 2005). Describing things as placebos is more likely than not to be similar to describing disease as an imbalance in the four humors or a consequence of inauspicious alignment of the stars. Placebo is a strange notion that has recently gained momentum in an ever expanding placebo literature. But more attention paid to placebo is no reason to think placebo is more worthy of attention, more substantial or more enduring.

5 Beecher's Placebo Revisited

Beecher's claim that placebos are powerful has suffered several powerful blows. Kienle and Kiene (1997) reviewed the trials on which Beecher based his conclusions. Their findings could hardly have been more opposite to his: "none of the original trials cited by Beecher gave grounds to assume the existence of placebo effects." They found no evidence of any placebo effects. They cataloged many alternative explanations, however, including errors, biases, statistical interpretation and spontaneous improvement.

Three systematic reviews of more recent trials also failed to find Beecher's powerful placebo. Hróbjartsson and Gøtzsche (2001, 2004, 2010) analyzed clinical trials comparing a placebo group with a no-treatment group:

> In general, placebo treatments produced no major health benefits, although on average they had a modest effect on outcomes reported by patients, such as pain. However, the effect on pain varied from large to non-existent, even in well-conducted trials. Variations in the effect of placebo was partly explained by variations in how trials were conducted, the type of placebo used, and whether patients were informed that the trial involved placebo (Hróbjartsson and Gøtzsche 2010).

These systematic reviews have been criticized (Wampold et al. 2005, Miller and Rosenstein 2006, Benedetti 2009). For instance,

Benedetti (2009) writes of the meta-analysis in 2001 by Hróbjartsson and Gøtzsche that "now most researchers do not take it very seriously" because the inclusion criteria were too broad while critical factors such as expectation and context were omitted, among other criticisms. Yet Benedetti's own placebo proposals raise questions, such as the tenuous expansion of placebo to include placebo-related effects in the absence of placebos.

After re-analyzing some of the same reports, Wampold et al. (2005) reassert the power of placebo as robust. Hróbjartsson and Gøtzsche (2007) counter that Wampold et al., "put powerful spin on their conclusion despite similar results as the original review." Miller and Rosenstein (2006) argue to the contrary that there is support for the reality of the placebo effect and call for more research, saying there is a difference between clinical trials that show weak or no placebo effect, because patients aren't told that the placebo is powerful, and clinical practice in which patients are told and believe the placebo is powerful and therefore show a greater placebo effect.

Meissner et al. (2007) examined some of the same trials reviewed by Hróbjartsson and Gøtzsche (2001, 2004) and by dividing the data into subgroups found that placebos can improve "physical parameters" (in diseases such as hypertension and asthma) but not "biochemical parameters" (in diseases such as diabetes and hypercholesterolaemia). They found these results in studies with or without a no-treatment group. They added this caution, however:

> Depending on the type of disease (e.g., psychiatric, neurological, internal), on the information delivered to the patient, and on the patient's former experiences with treatments, the effects of placebo interventions may differ, and different mechanisms may be involved. To disentangle the specific components of placebo treatments under different circumstances and to work out their effects represents a major challenge for future placebo research.

Here we see again the all-encompassing domain of placebo that is said to range over different types of diseases, interventions and mechanisms. In particular it is important to distinguish the levels of analysis and organization of proposed mechanisms. Neurotransmitters, conditioning, learning, coping, adaptation, anxiety, belief, hope, expectation and context are not all at the same levels. To say what the boundaries of those levels are and how the levels interact is an intractable exercise.

These examples typify the back-and-forth of science, in which the usual aim is to choose the best among the rest, so I must emphasize that the relevance of these studies to this discussion is not to decide which ones are right but rather to show how all sides are struggling within the current placebo paradigm to express a coherent conception of placebo. The sides could not be much more polarized. At one extreme we have the received wisdom of Beecher's powerful placebo effect while at the other extreme is little or no evidence of placebo effects in systematic reviews of many trials. In between are various compromises, such as saying there is not one placebo effect but many different placebo effects. Placebos are a real phenomenon for some and an illusion for others.

Infancy of placebo research

Placebo problems have been apparent since the placebo concept was introduced. Like many researchers who have subsequently found or failed to find evidence of his powerful placebo, Beecher (1955) was less interested in terminological or theoretical questions than about practical use of placebos for their effects in clinical situations. Yet he too noted that the term placebo was inadequate: "If it falls a bit short of precision, perhaps the language will have to grow a little..." Now more than a half-century later, we remain constrained by that lack of precision.

Having reviewed various placebo experiments, Enck et al. (2008) conclude with the question, "Where Does Placebo Research Go from Here?" This excerpt from their answer is revealing:

> Despite the recent explosion of neurobiological placebo research using sophisticated tools, such as neuroimaging, in vivo receptor binding, and single-neuron recording in awake subjects, our knowledge of the mechanisms underlying the placebo effect is still in its infancy, and several issues need to be addressed in future research. The major questions to be answered are where, when, how, and why placebo effects occur. In fact, we need to know where they work exactly, that is, in which medical conditions. For example, are all diseases and symptoms subject to placebo effects? We also need to know when they work, that is, whether there are special circumstances that are particularly amenable to placebo effects. How they work is also a major question, as we need to understand the brain mechanisms at both the macroscopic (brain regions and their interactions with body functions) and microscopic (cellular and molecular) level. Finally, determining why placebo effects exist at all represents a major scientific challenge, and meeting that challenge will give us insights into the possible evolution of endogenous healthcare systems.

They begin by referring to the infancy of placebo knowledge and say several issues need to be addressed, as is common in research, but then they list major unanswered questions that have defied those engaged in the current engrained placebo research program. This suggests that it's not only the infancy of the research program that limits placebo knowledge, but the problem is also the complex intractable placebo concept itself that prevents the infant from developing into a mature adult no matter how much more data from brain studies it feeds on.

Are brain mechanisms placebo mechanisms?

With the availability of computerized brain imaging technology, current research dictates that the most persuasive evidence of placebo effects will be found in the brain. The reasoning goes something like this: If a treatment that only resembles real treatment appears to have biological effects (and to be really persuasive, also has correlated changes in the brain) then placebos have real biological effects and therefore placebo is a real biological phenomenon.

Many different mechanisms in the brain have been proposed to explain and control placebo effects including dopamine, endogenous opioids, serotonin, oxytocin, nitric oxide and cholecystokynin among others. These neuro-level mechanisms have been explored using a variety of treatments for different conditions. Proponents of the neuroscientific placebo research program point to these mechanisms as the final source of answers to questions about placebo effects:

> We are witnessing an epochal passage, when purely theoretical entities like 'suggestibility' and 'power of the mind' are finally being replaced by biological accuracy and molecular certainty, with rituals and context interpreted in terms of specific brain regions and biochemical pathways activated. The capacity of the mind to affect the body can now become visible and mechanistically understandable... (Pollo et al. 2011).

Seeing is believing when it comes to brain mechanisms perhaps, but that does not mean brain mechanisms will empirically drive out all theoretical devils. To say they are mechanisms of placebo effects is to preserve the mysterious theoretical entities called placebo and placebo effects.

Both pain and Parkinson's disease, for instance. have been treated experimentally with placebo, nocebo, verbal suggestion and open versus hidden drug administration. From these experiments, the mechanism said to be associated with pain has been summarized as, "Expectation-induced activation of endogenous opioids and cholecystokinin as well as of several brain regions" while the mechanism associated with Parkinson's disease has been summarized as "Expectation-induced release of dopamine in the striatum and changes of firing pattern of subthalamic nucleus neurons" (Benedetti 2008). Another way of describing the mechanisms elucidated in Parkinson's disease is as "reward-related mechanisms" based on associations between reward, motivation and the regions of the brain that respond (de la Fuente-Fernández and Stoessl 2002). Each postulated mechanism involves various levels, such as the psychological levels of expectation, reward and motivation together with the neurochemical levels of opioids and dopamine.

One way of demonstrating these mechanisms is by intervening to turn them on and off. For example, the opioid antagonist naloxone can be administered to interfere with endogenous opioids and turn off placebo analgesia. If experimenters can control the brain's placebo mechanisms like switching lights on and off at will, doesn't that make sense of placebo? Why abandon the notion of placebo now that these placebo mechanisms have been demonstrated experimentally?

For mechanisms to make sense of placebo, we have to make sense of mechanisms. Yet there is no general agreement about mechanisms in medicine or in science. It's not clear what is meant by saying that dopamine, reward or expectation is a placebo mechanism. Clearly it's not a mechanism like a lever or a cog in any machine manufactured and acceptable for use by humans. Properly engineered levers and cogs don't fail to work in a large majority of their machines the way placebos fail to work in most people. Yet if Beecher was right, placebo mechanisms fail in the majority of observed cases.

The claim that expectation is a placebo mechanism cannot be as strong as a claim that there is a law of nature, like the law of gravity, such that patients with particular expectations show placebo effects. Does that mean the language of mechanism is used to avoid talking of medicine in terms of natural laws? Or if there is such a law of placebo expectation, albeit one involving considerable uncertainty, what explains individual variation and exceptions to the law? If the expectation mechanism of placebo is not an expression of general law, is the mechanism always present or does it come and go, and if so how long does the mechanism have to operate to be effective? If there is no regularity, it's difficult to see what role placebo mechanisms play in explaining placebo and placebo effects.

This should be no surprise given that placebo mechanisms are said to be many things at mixed conceptual levels, mental and physical, psychological and chemical, individual and social. Mechanism in relation to medicine typically is limited to the search for the specific mechanism responsible for a specific condition, such as finding the mechanism that will stop the patient's pain. But considering mechanisms at the level of the social sciences, Astbury and Leeuw (2010) situate placebo among "belief-formation mechanisms" that "have been used to explain a variety of social phenomena, such as hypnosis; placebo and Hawthorne effects; the failure of banks and stock market crashes; and the processes of racial and religious prejudice."

The idea of mechanism invokes broad issues such as how to define mechanism, the relative importance of distinguishing how something works from why it works, whether talk of mechanism is a substitute for talk of scientific laws and how a mechanism view can handle reduction and emergence in different levels of organization.

In a widely cited analysis of mechanisms in neurobiology and molecular biology, Machamer et al. (2000) propose a broad, abstract conception of the role of mechanisms in explanation:

"Mechanisms are entities and activities organized such that they are productive of regular changes from start or set-up to finish or termination conditions." Such regular changes could include the statistical regularities currently labeled as placebo effects. Bunge (2004) rejects that definition as imprecise and incorrect, preferring to link mechanism to process, and as an aside states that, "placebos are mechanisms, since they trigger physiological processes that start in the cortex and may involve the release of neurotransmitters." So from this view placebos themselves are mechanisms, as distinct from the mechanisms of placebo. Given the uncertainty associated with placebo effects and placebo responders, it seems strange to say that placebos are productive of regular changes or that sugar pills become triggers that in most cases do not appear to have any observable medical outcome.

Are placebos mechanisms constituted of other mechanisms like a mechanical clock composed of wheels turning other wheels and dials? If placebos are mechanisms by virtue of triggering physiological processes, then conceivably everything encountered by humans is a mechanism linked to a placebo mechanism. An example of this broad view is the biopsychosocial Ethnomedicogenic Thesis of Hahn and Kleinman (1983) who describe the causal mechanism of placebo and nocebo in these terms: "...in a dialectical process, ethnomedical systems of belief and expectation causally affect the reality of sickness and health with efficacy perceptually reinforcing the referring ethnomedical system."

If mechanism is so broadly construed to include almost every imaginable part and composite of parts, and perhaps even wholes, then what is explained by casting expectation or anything else as mediator or mechanism of placebo? Expectation may be conceived as a mechanism, especially by those who think nothing is explained without mechanisms, but why cast it as a placebo mechanism? Is placebo an emergent property or epiphenomenon of proposed placebo mechanisms such as expectation or neurochemistry? Absent the notion of placebo, these placebo-related questions disappear: an observed improvement in a patient, together with brain correlates and other observations, may be described in terms of expectation and neurochemistry, or more likely a network of entities and processes, which may have their own mechanisms, perhaps recursively related all the way down.

Returning to the metaphor of a light switch, clearly a placebo mechanism is not the same notion as the deterministic mechanism of an electrical switch that either turns on the light, turns off the light or is broken. It's hard to say when a placebo mechanism works or is broken. Only some people respond to placebo at the best of times, so any talk of placebo mechanisms refers to frustratingly probabilistic ones. Placebo mechanisms apparently refer to observed differences within and between people, not to people as all-alike assembly-line mechanisms composed of clockwork sub-mechanisms.

Are placebo mechanisms more than a reflection of the methodologies used to elicit observations associated by a narrative under the title of placebo? To create a sensible narrative explaining even one concept such as an expectation mechanism, more than one explanation of the mechanism itself is required to integrate the various levels from neurochemistry to psychology to society. It's not clear, then, what pain and Parkinson's disease have in common that merits their association within the placebo narrative. They are not associated with the same physical divisions in brain or body, or similar subjective experiences, or neurochemistry. Parkinson's disease is considered to be an identifiable neurological movement disorder while pain is not associated with one disease, disorder or function, nor is it limited to one brain region or bodily system. To group pain and Parkinson's disease in the same placebo box is to mix concepts and conceptual levels, from neurochemistry to psychological constructs including expectation, reward and conditioning, to the varied mixture of things associated with placebo such as context, meaning, fake drugs, surgery and words.

If instead the placebo layer were omitted, then these interventions would not be conceived as placebo mechanisms. For the materialist reductionist, perhaps they would all be brain mechanisms. Others may talk in terms of higher levels and emergent features not reducible to the brain. In any case they would not be placebo mechanisms. For example, if dopamine is deemed to be a mechanism in Parkinson's disease, not a placebo mechanism, then it could be said that patients with Parkinson's disease sometimes can be conditioned and their expectations may sometimes be altered in various ways, while correlated changes in dopamine and patient symptoms can be measured.

While a substance such as dopamine could be viewed as a brain mechanism in biomedical experiments, it's less clear what to make of the psychological constructs of expectation and conditioning when they are gathered with dopamine as kinds of placebo mechanisms. With respect to the different problem of understanding pain, endogenous opioids can be measured and correlated with conditioning, learning, anxiety, expectation and other influences on reported pain. But not only is this an unruly mixture of substances, such as dopamine and opioids, with psychology, in constructs such as conditioning and expectation, but measures of dopamine in Parkinson's disease and opioids in pain experiments are the consequences of different interventions in different contexts in different experiments on different people with different conditions.

Do these purported placebo mechanisms unify ideas and show simple relationships, generalizations and laws that explain apparently disparate phenomena? The brief summaries quoted above suggest a relationship called expectation-related or reward-related mediators of placebo effects. But that can't be an adequate description, since expectation-related doesn't account for the conditioning involved in experiments with Parkinson's disease, or for conditioning that influences expectation. Nor could an expression such as expectation-conditioning-reward-related or any other committee-constructed camel improve our understanding of what is observed. No single expression is adequate to tie these experiments together, and placebo certainly doesn't do the trick.

We gain little from entangling pain and Parkinson's disease, and their associated brain regions and neurochemistry, together with psychological constructs such as expectation, reward and conditioning, and social constructs such as meaning and context, in the impossible knot called placebo or placebo mediator or placebo mechanism or placebo effect. Recent neurobiological discoveries cannot resolve traditional confusions about placebo but can only graft more dichotomies and epicycles on a placebo-centric conception of the universe.

6 Placebo Reality Check

In discussions of placebo, notions of *real* and *reality* may be wielded in different ways and in reference to different things. Real may refer to medical conditions, symptoms, treatments and observed effects among other possibilities. Symptoms are often divided between the real or the imagined: it's not real, it's all in your head. In this regard, the question has often been raised whether placebos cure real diseases or are just in the imagination of patients and medical providers. Or the division could be real versus malingering: it's not just the placebo that's fake, the patient is presenting a fake problem.

Talk of imagination and personal experience raises questions of subjectivity and phenomenology: can placebo be understood by third-party observers or are answers to placebo questions limited to the realm of first-person explorations? Talk of malingering also raises issues of objectivity: can patient fakery be exposed by, for instance, brain scans comparing the brains of fakers with those of genuine cases? Talk of real diseases raises questions of classification and social construction. Some would say that the word real cannot apply to disease at all, as diseases are social constructs that change with time and medical fashion. From that viewpoint no disease can be called real. Talk of real effects leads to distinctions between real placebo effects and other effects that might be confused with what is real.

Placebos themselves are defined in terms of reality, as placebos are often said to be fake not real treatments. In biomedicine, the distinction may be that a real treatment has some physical content, a chemical property or a surgical procedure, that does the work. Placebo effects, like placebos, are also defined by their reality.

Placebo reality is bound up with related concepts of truth, objectivity and fact. Are placebos and their effects objective scientific facts, if indeed any objective facts exist, or are they aspects of a reality constructed by people who think of the world in terms of placebos? Answers depend in part on whether placebo is deemed to be an observable thing, such as a pill, or a process, such as a response to a meaningful experience, or an artifact, such as a change in a brain image. The reality of observable placebo pills is a different issue than the reality of unobservable placebo processes or their traces made visible.

Ultimate questions hover over matters such as whether we can ever know what is real and true or approximately true. Consider a few droplets from an ocean of musings about these issues. According to Charles S. Peirce in his frequently quoted essay of 1878, *How To Make Our Ideas Clear*, reality is a matter of opinion: "The opinion which is fated to be ultimately agreed to by all who investigate, is what we mean by the truth, and the object represented in this opinion is the real. That is the way I would explain reality."

Albert Einstein (1938) famously wrote that, "In our endeavour to understand reality we are somewhat like a man trying to understand the mechanism of a closed watch. He sees the face and the moving hands, even hears its ticking, but he has no way of opening the case... He will never be able to compare his picture with the real mechanism and he cannot even imagine the possibility or the meaning of such a comparison."

Ludwick Fleck (1979) in his seminal work *Genesis and Development of a Scientific Fact* called truth, "(1) in historical perspective, an event in the history of thought, (2) in its contemporary perspective, stylized thought constraint." For Fleck, a scientific fact is the product of a collective community of thinkers, "the signal of resistance opposing free, arbitrary thinking." If Fleck were to ask a scientist why we have the conception we now have of placebo, the answer might be: because it is true or approximately true. Yet in historical and cultural perspective, the various incarnations of placebo, let alone the various cultural traditions that do not even have a notion of placebo, appear to be mutually incommensurable and cannot all stand for the same facts and truths. It is not enough simply to distinguish real or true placebo effects from something else.

The point for this discussion is not to digress into an attempt to resolve these difficult conceptual problems concerning reality and truth in general, which would take us far from a discussion of placebo, but only to maintain vigilance about the various expressions of the real and true in relation to placebo and placebo effects.

Problematic placebo theory

Theories and hypotheses that have become encrusted around the term placebo share problems inherent in all theories of science and medicine. An overriding problem is the difficulty of formulating any theories at all in medicine. Philosopher Paul Tang (1999) questions whether there can ever be scientific theories in psychology, medicine, or psychiatry. He examines a typical placebo-controlled experiment and concludes that the science is too rudimentary to provide rigorous theories.

At the other extreme are those who expect medical theories to be like theories in physics and chemistry. For instance, one prominent theory of health considers it to be a value-free, objective matter of natural science and statistics (Boorse 1976, 1977). But even the basic sciences, including the princely science of physics, cannot escape many problems debated by philosophers of science, such as the absence of a purely empirical method for choosing between competing beliefs and theories, or a way to translate terms across competing world views and theories, or any assurance that present observations and theories are stable given the instability of past theories.

Consider several basic models of placebo, starting with the bare-bones version introduced earlier:

Placebos cause placebo effects.

This statement seems to be asserting something meaningful. But if this is not to be seen as a tautology, we have to assume all sorts of things about these words, perhaps that placebos are fake treatments and that placebo effects are observed improvements in the conditions of patients taking placebos. Ignore for now the subtleties of the word cause, and ignore also the mysteries underlying a statement about placebos causing anything while being fake or inert, and ignore any concerns about which improvements are attributable to placebo. The best that can be said about placebos causing placebo effects, as for most medical interventions, is that some patients get better and some don't. Although estimates vary widely, no serious estimate asserts that placebos always work in everyone. So the statement must be revised to include uncertainty:

Placebos may cause placebo effects.

Now the statement is weak and verging on meaningless. If a placebo treatment is associated with improvement in only 35% of the studied population, as Beecher famously reported, what were the other 65% doing? The uncertainty of medicine may excuse our lack of understanding of medical treatments, including placebos.

But the uncertainty excuse is not an explanation of what is happening, either in those who respond to placebos or those who don't respond. The usual failure of some patients to respond to treatment, including placebo treatment, is not considered to negate placebo theory. That placebos most often do not work is no proof that placebos never work. Yet by incorporating uncertainty in our statement about placebo effects, we have less certainty about the whole matter of placebo.

Organisms are moving targets always changing over time, so medicine is always *in media res*, and explanations in medicine are not typically stories of starting and stopping but only of influencing ongoing processes. Even birth and death are not medical starts and stops but involve ongoing relationships among living entities and between individuals and their environments. There is, for instance, no way to observe the exact instant when life is extinguished. Patients are not machines or physics experiments that can be constructed, switched on, tested, switched off and reconstructed to repeat the same experiment. Distinguishing what would have happened in the story from what eventually happens adds particular complexity to medicine.

Natural course of disease is one explanation for what may appear to be placebo effects: a person who takes a placebo gets better not because of the placebo but because the natural course of the disease over time for that person in the circumstances is to get better. Now we have two statements to integrate:

Placebos may cause placebo effects.

Natural course of disease may account for what appear to be placebo effects.

This seems sensible, that the body and its diseases have a natural course or natural history. Time makes a difference. What then is natural course or history? Let's say for a moment that natural course is a homeostatic or allostatic response by the body to disease such that, when its course is undisturbed, returns the person to a state without the disease or as near as possible in the circumstances. With chronic disease, natural course may be an adaptive response that does something less than eliminate the disease entirely. Or perhaps in a broader sense natural course is the self-repair that distinguishes living from non-living things: rocks can't fix themselves but rabbits can, and robots may some day soon repair and reproduce themselves and claim entry to the ranks of the living.

But can we ever know what that natural course is in any individual case? And whether we can or not, is any person's actual history ever natural in the sense of being undisturbed by other factors? Natural course, like placebo, is more a description of effects observed in the absence of other things, that is, self-cure effects, than a meaningful expression of what causes the effects. Consider these possibilities:

—The natural course of disease could be equated with what happens in untreated people: natural course equals no treatment. But with respect to placebo, are any individuals actually untreated? That is, if the concept of placebo includes and is relevant to any medical intervention, then almost anything a person experiences acts as a placebo (or nocebo if the effect is unwanted) and interferes with the natural course. Only individuals who have no contact with substances, procedures, words, symbols, meanings, people or ideas that might influence belief, expectation, hope or other relevant matters, are untreated by placebos.

—For those who accept that the mind or brain has some direct influence on health and disease, the natural course of disease includes mental as well as physical processes. How is natural course differentiated between mind (or brain) and body? Placebo theory is modeled on mental processes such as expectation and belief. It's hard to tell the difference between an untreated mental process that influences disease and a placebo process.

—Also problematic is the notion of measuring the natural course. Any method claiming to be scientific needs to measure things, but measurement of natural course requires some interaction with the person. Because almost any interaction can be a placebo, then almost any kind of measurement could by itself be considered to act as a placebo. Perhaps measurements of which the person is unconscious would not be considered to be placebo treatment, if such measurement were practically and ethically possible. In any event, theories of placebo derived from unconscious or experimentally manufactured measurements are unlikely to apply in the typical medical context in which informed consent is required.

—Natural course need not be considered synonymous with lack of treatment. If the underlying nature that cures a person operates continuously in any person whether treated or untreated, then the natural course would be operating in patients who receive treatment but do not respond to treatment. But still the question remains how to disentangle the natural course from the course of treatment.

Given the broad inclusiveness of the placebo notion, natural course is not clearly separable from what are now called placebo effects. Nor is natural course an adequate explanation for the distinction between placebo cure and self-cure in the absence of placebo. Subtle distinctions can be made among related terms such as natural course, natural history, self-healing, self-cure, spontaneous remission, spontaneous regression, autonomous response and many others. For instance, remission could mean getting better, regression could describe statistical artifacts, and autonomous response could mean any response whether getting better or worse or autonomously suffering from additional problems. But the puzzle remains of integrating these possibilities with placebo, placebo effects and people.

Some medical problems seem to appear and disappear as symptoms fluctuate. People often become patients when their symptoms worsen to the point that they seek help. At that low point they get tested and measured by their physicians. Later measurements appear to regress toward their mean value. Other fluctuations, including many chronic effects of aging, become everyday adaptations as the person changes. Familiar aches and pains of aging and chronic disease that once may have prompted a visit to the doctor may be deemed by the suffering person no longer to require medical intervention.

How can we parse the natural course of a person's history into these and other time-related components of self-adjustment and accommodation, fluctuating symptoms and statistical artifacts? Placebo-controlled trials usually compare an experimental treatment group with a placebo control group. They rarely include an additional control group, the so-called no-treatment group. The idea behind a no-treatment control is to compare the placebo with no treatment. Give some people a fake pill or procedure, give other people nothing and see if the fake works better than nothing. If the fake does work better, perhaps then we can conclude that fake pills and procedures are powerful.

Unlike the typical placebo-controlled trial in which a placebo is used as the control, with a no-treatment group the placebo is also deemed to be a kind of treatment while its control is doing nothing, letting nature take its course. Although this kind of comparison is occasionally made, one problem is the simple linear assumption that any two contexts of treatment or no treatment can be subtracted (or added). Instead they may have complex non-linear relations with feedback and other dynamic features better understood from a complexity-theoretical view.

Placebo obscures complexity

Science proceeds by reducing complex entities into things that can be tested and controlled separately. A medical outcome, however, depends on many things that interact with many other things and these many-to-many interactions spawn a combinatorial explosion of complexity.

One classification of these many things connected to many other things follows from the common idea that medical symptoms must have causes that produce effects through various mechanisms operating over a span of time. Each instance within each category (symptom, cause, effect, mechanism, time) connects to many possibilities, at various levels ranging from the subatomic to the social, with many symptoms, causes, mechanisms, effects and times connecting to many other things.

We do not build simple linear models for a weather forecast by saying some proportion of sun and wind added to some proportion of cloud and moisture sums up to future observed weather. We rely instead on sophisticated dynamical mathematical models of weather implemented in computer software running on supercomputers. Medical models should be at least as sophisticated as weather models. But placebo is often modeled as a linear one-to-one relation such as:

placebo + drug = outcome

or from the point of view of psychological mechanisms:

expectation + conditioning = placebo response

Such linear models ignore concepts of sensitivity to initial conditions, non-linear dynamics, self-reference and feedback among interacting network nodes that appear in complex systems.

In a complexity-theoretical view, components cannot be modeled like the addition and subtraction of simple mechanical forces.

A patient who guesses that the pill is a placebo may respond not only to the pill but also to the patient's own expectation of how patients respond to placebo pills and how guesses relate to actuality. Expectation may involve an expectation of an expectation, a second-order or meta-expectation, about how we expect to behave given our expectations and experiences of our own expectation-induced actions. How would I feel if I drank a cup of coffee without knowing whether it contained caffeine? Would that be a different feeling than if I knew how much caffeine it contained? How would I expect to feel if the dentist were to start drilling into my tooth after a placebo injection? Merely asking the question can cause a reaction.

Self-referencing entities such as expectation are not linear or statically additive but non-linear and dynamic. The map of expectation might include not only patient expectations of other patients taking similar pills but also provider expectations of what the pill provider might expect of patients generally and of this person in particular. Or regardless of expectation, the effects of some biomedical treatments might be detectable only in the presence of other factors that are not generally considered to be causal in biomedicine, such as enthusiasm.

Furthermore, within the realm of self-expectation are variations. Expectations of one's own response to a treatment, such as feeling pain, can be distinguished from stimulus expectancies, such as the expectation of good grades on an examination (Kirsch 1999). The student does not control what grades the teacher reports, whereas grading and reporting of one's own pain are within one's own sphere of influence. Expectation of pain relief may lead to a self-fulfilling non-volitional response perceived as pain relief.

Self-referent feedback models are far removed from linear models of placebo causing placebo effects added to or subtracted from a notional natural course. Perhaps the feedback recurses repeatedly, as when one expects oneself to expect a response from oneself, which expectation and response further influence the response. Humans are actively gaming the system, trying to figure out what's happening, how the game is run and why and whether it is worth playing, continually testing the process, assessing their options and the consequences.

To note the kind of oversimplification that the placebo notion facilitates is not to argue against the traditional scientific practice of taking things apart, reducing them to individual factors then trying to rebuild them and control them. Rather it is to say that we can't only look at neuromechanisms or any other individual mechanisms or parts. If everything can be reduced to the lowest level then have the higher levels nothing to offer? Conversely, if only a holistic overall view provides answers, then do the ingredients that comprise the whole have nothing to contribute? We have to consider various levels of analysis and of physical organization, from brain chemistry to individual to society not only apart but also together in dynamic non-linear many-to-many interactions. To do so demands not a placebo view but a non-linear complexity view, together with appropriate methodologies.

A non-linear complexity view of medicine with a possibly chaotic non-deterministic network conception rather than a deterministic linear continuum could free placebo researchers from the chains of thinking in pairs. In medicine after placebo, we might get beyond false dichotomies such as mind-body, active-inert, specific-non-specific, subjective-objective and so on. Placebo-free language may lead to dichotomy-reduced language.

Placebo disposed

Many observations could be cast into effect language as medical observations have been cast into placebo effects: puddles in the street are rain effects, babies are sexual intercourse effects and laughter at stand-up comedy is a performer or audience effect. It's easier to talk of effects than causes. Causal networks can be difficult to untangle. The causes of your existence, for instance, are not just events involving your parents but include events going back in historical, evolutionary and cosmic time. Your birth and your subsequent health or disease are conditional effects of countless events that happened to line up in a particular way.

One way to frame placebo from the viewpoint of effects is to talk of dispositional properties or powers. Unlike substantial, categorical, observable properties such as size, dispositional properties are unobservable properties that describe the disposition, potential, power or capacity to cause some effect. Dispositional properties describe what something can do if some other conditions arise. If the conditions actually arise, the disposition is manifested in some event.

A common example is fragility. A glass window has the disposition to break. Fragility is manifested in the effect of breaking. Although the glass may break into pieces when hit by a hammer, its fragility is not an observable property like its size. The fragility of glass doesn't become apparent unless certain conditions are met, such as hitting the glass sufficiently hard with a hammer. Another common example of a disposition is solubility: for instance, sugar is disposed to dissolve in water. Dispositions are ascribed not only to things and types of things but also to people, as for instance when someone is said to have a pleasant disposition or is disposed to be generous.

Some theorists assert that without dispositional properties, we cannot account for our experience of the world while others say that dispositional properties are unnecessary fictions. The latter viewpoint parallels the present thesis about placebo: nothing is gained by introducing the intermediate category of placebo between cause and effect. To review the many debated issues about dispositional properties would be major a digression if pursued here, including whether dispositional properties are categorical properties by another name, or are dependent on categorical properties, or whether any properties are not dispositional. For the purposes of this discussion, a dispositional view illuminates further concerns about the notion of placebo.

Placebos seem to fit into a dispositional view since they are expressed in terms of the effects they cause, namely placebo effects. So it seems as if placebos have dispositions, powers, propensities, capacities or whatever term expresses their capability to cause placebo effects. Placebo effects do not appear in all contexts but only in conditional, iffy contexts.

Just as the fragility of glass becomes manifest in certain effects that might be observed as cracking or shattering, it could be said that the disposition of sugar pills to cure becomes manifest when given to patients who believe that the pills are powerful drugs. The dispositional medicinal powers of sugar are conditional and manifest themselves only in some contexts. Of course this is vacuously circular reasoning: sugar consumed in other contexts that don't show placebo effects would not attract the placebo label.

The power of placebo sugar seems to be in its non-specificity for biomedical effects, not like its invisibility when dissolved in water. Placebo sugar manifests its placebo power in a much broader range of medical circumstances and observations than its solubility power, if there are such powers. A placebo sugar pill that relieves a headache manifests its power as pain reduction whereas a placebo sugar pill in a study of cardiac medication might be observed to influence blood pressure. The placebo power of sugar, unlike its relatively narrow power of solubility, appears to be unbounded; apparently placebo sugar can manifest its power in all of medicine. Perhaps then it's a mistake to say that placebo sugar has medicinal power in the same way that ordinary sugar has the power to dissolve. One might argue that it's better to say the power to dissolve is in the sugar but placebo power is in the person.

From such metaphysical distinctions one could write a library of placebo literature. A dispositional view of sugar pills, and other medical interventions that seem to have dispositions or powers that become observable as placebo effects, would no doubt lead to fine distinctions that could fuel further debate. The approach here is to leave the metaphysical debate over dispositions or powers to metaphysicians and instead to eliminate the placebo notion for clinical physicians and medical researchers.

No magic placebo bullet

Many questions surface in the context of placebo causes and effects including: what do we mean when we say something is the cause or cure of a disease, what is the standard of evidence required to establish a causal connection, how much uncertainty should we accept when drawing causal conclusions and making decisions, and ultimately whether a causal explanation is even possible.

In David Hume's skeptical epistemology, which is often taken as the starting point for considering problems of causation, the best we can observe is constant conjunctions or connections we deem necessary. Causation for Hume and sympathetic empiricists is such a problem that many would say the search for causes should be abandoned. A Humean gaze removes the causal story of placebo, or how the causal story of medical treatments is connected to the unknown causal story of placebo. This accords with the empiricist methods of evidence-based medicine and the randomized placebo-controlled trials that, despite claims to causal explanation, merely track conjunctions between interventions and outcomes.

At the opposite extreme lies specific etiology, and more specifically germ theory, in which diseases are identifiable things separable from the body and demonstrably caused by specific mechanisms, namely germs. According to Koch's well-known postulates, preventing or curing disease is reducible to finding and removing a single necessary, if not sufficient, cause. Hand-washing removes bacteria that cause disease so hand-washing is a way to prevent disease caused by bacteria. But this simple magic-bullet theory ignores many complexities, including whether diseases are strictly identifiable things, and whether they and the body can be separated from each other and their environment. A succinct summary is provided by psychiatrist Herbert Spiegel (1997):

> With Pasteur's discovery of bacteria, biological reductionism became the pathway for medicine to develop into a scientific discipline. Causes of diseases could be analyzed into single identifiable parts, which could then be specifically targeted and treated. Dazzling achievements ensued in the cure and prevention of bacterial diseases. The record of success has had the effect of convincing the mainstream of medicine that biological reductionism is the only appropriate approach to understanding and coping with health and disease. Yet this paradigm has not yielded the same measure of success in the treatment of illnesses related to aging, allergies, immune diseases, and cancer as it has with bacterial diseases.

Despite its obvious oversimplification, germ theory remains central to medicine and is one of the foundations of the current focus on genetics and individualized medicine.

The Hill criteria have become another vigorously debated standard for assessing medical causation. Hill (1965) set out nine indicia of causation, what he called aspects and viewpoints, to consider before concluding that an observed association is causal. They are: strength, consistency, specificity, temporality, biological gradient, plausibility, coherence, experiment and analogy. All of these terms have been debated. Specificity is especially problematic for placebo, which in some expositions is what remains, the non-specific effects, after accounting for specificity. In what sense can the specificity of a non-specific effect be specified? In this regard, placebo can be viewed as the background not the causal foreground.

Hume, Koch and Hill represent only a part of the vast landscape of theorizing about causation in medicine. The placebo notion adds the difficulty of accounting for associations between fake treatment, observations and events in the mind, or brain, together with associated questions about causal connections between the mind and the world.

Placebo doesn't fit any ordinary causal theory of disease or cure. It's not a specific magic bullet that kills a specific pathogen. It has no power of its own to kill germs. It is not an antidote to specific or general poisons. It is consistent with both an external germ-causes-disease theory and an internal disease-is-in-the-body theory, in which the placebo may have observed effects without regard to causes, or with vague nods to something going on between mind or brain and body.

No placebo nothing

In common comparisons between a drug and a placebo, the placebo is often considered to represent doing nothing. Even the renowned clinical trial pioneer Austin Bradford Hill (1963) refers to placebo as nothing. But if a placebo is a nothing treatment, it's confusing to speak of experimentally comparing placebo nothing with no-treatment nothing. It's impossible in practice to study someone inertly. No absolute placebo effect can be measured against an absolute no-treatment group. Only a relative comparison is possible between the fake treatment group and whatever is specified as the self-aware, self-treated, no-treatment group.

Such groups are many. They could conceivably be among the following examples:

—placebo (fake drug or procedure)
—placebo that mimics side effects ("active placebo")
—alternative treatment (with or without placebo add-on)
—no treatment (with consent, perhaps on a waiting list)
—no contact (no consent, unaware of being studied)

Of these groups, the no-contact group comes closest to the purity of the imaginary perfect experimental control, the purely no-treatment group. The no-contact group, however, spied upon while unaware of being studied, would be difficult to justify in most circumstances under present ethical rules. Only if we could put the same people in two parallel universes or rewind the clock and run the experiment again would we have exactly equal groups, *ceteris paribus*, but for being treated or not treated. All practical groups are compromises among various methodological and ethical values.

Various practical solutions to the no-treatment problem have been suggested, including the waiting-list group or a statistical study. One solution could be to redefine no-treatment to mean no-treatment among other treatments. For instance in a study of pain, three groups could get the same analgesic but one group could receive additional treatment and another group could receive fake additional treatment. Is the difference between the two add-on groups a meaningful difference between fake and real treatment? No group in this example is a no-treatment group. The measured difference between add-on groups cannot account for the complexity of interactions among the treatments. No completely satisfactory no-treatment condition is possible.

Observing patients has been compared to the Heisenberg uncertainty relation in physics and the Hawthorne effect in social science (Hróbjartsson 1996). The physics metaphor expresses the idea that to measure particles is to move them, so that for instance measuring a particle's momentum changes its position. The social science metaphor expresses the idea that studying people influences their behavior, so that for instance the act of interviewing workers without actually improving working conditions could nevertheless make them feel better about their workplace. Experimenters do not merely observe but also influence what is observed.

Participants who do not receive treatment, and who may only be names on a waiting list, are still special participants in an experiment who have contacts with experimenters, who consent to be on the list and who know they are on a list that is being monitored by experts. To the extent that perceived control influences medical outcomes, merely stating in a consent form that the person may freely withdraw consent could increase perceived control and influence the outcome (Rosnow and Rosenthal 1997). Consent alone can distinguish experimental subjects from the general population and therefore bias experimental outcomes.

Experimental subjects may give their consent for many reasons ranging from general beliefs in altruism to specific need for drugs. Beecher (1970) succinctly states the consequence of consent for any volunteer human experiments. After examining the many motives and personal attributes associated with volunteers in experiments, he concludes that, "the use of volunteers alone may give a false picture of the general population." Waiting-list participants are specially identified, voluntary participants distinguished from the general population. Context effects may appear to be greater in identified than anonymous participants (Silverman 1968).

In some instances, more is done to the waiting-list group than mere waiting. Asking participants if they smoke, for example, could influence smoking behavior, or a baseline fitness assessment could influence eating and exercising behavior. A waiting list also implies that they are waiting for something. The presence of interested experts, the hope, the expectation, the possibility of treatment after the waiting period, these and related themes can distinguish people on the waiting list from people who have received no interest and who have no attentive experts eager to learn about the effects of no treatment on them.

The context of an experiment, quite apart from treatment, is not equivalent to doing nothing. Expectations, conditioning and other explanations of placebo effects can be associated with a no-treatment group. Moerman (2002) puts it this way: "except under the most extraordinary circumstances it is logically and conceptually impossible to have a no-treatment group."

Jopling (2008), however, says Moerman's concerns are too absolute, and that there is a continuum of greater or lesser treatment that can be informative. But pragmatically relaxing the requirements for a no-treatment group does not change the conceptual problems inherent when experimenting on humans. In addition, for medical conditions that have an effective treatment, withholding that treatment and using a no-treatment group instead would generally be considered unethical.

Any no-treatment experiment is a conceptual creation that predetermines the answer to the question what is no treatment and what is placebo. Does a no-treatment group include people whose family members offer support and encouragement, or just isolated individuals without family? Does a no-treatment group ignore changes in self-talk, diet, or other treatment given to oneself in light of one's assessment of one's own medical condition? Such a move would imply that placebo effects exclude self-treatment effects. When you are awake in bed at night, and thinking about your symptoms, and telling yourself that you'll feel better in the morning, is that thinking and telling considered to be no treatment? Is there no power of suggestion in self-talk? If you don't think at all about your own medical condition, is that considered to be no treatment or is it a pathological condition to be treated? What if you get up in the night for a glass of water to make yourself feel better, perhaps in response to seeing a poster about the health benefits of hydration at the clinic where you signed the consent for a clinical trial; is that treatment? Who never self-prescribes over-the-counter medications that have been recommended by some authorities yet failed to demonstrate efficacy in clinical trials, as for instance remedies for the common cold? Self-medication with recommended treatments in the no-treatment group resembles placebo treatment given by experimenters to the placebo group. It is difficult to conceive of a value-free, naturally occurring no-treatment state. A pure do-nothing control is a pure fiction.

Placebo people

Returning now to the basic description of placebo and placebo effects, let's add the people in whom effects are observed. The statement:

Placebos may cause placebo effects.

could therefore be extended to include the observed people as well as the effects:

Placebos may cause placebo effects in some people.

From this we might infer that a special kind of person, the placebo responder, differs from other people. Now the statement recognizes the possibility that medical conditions are not influenced only by things outside the person but also by things internal to the individual or type of person.

We could also add other actors such as treatment providers along with various other elements that for brevity could be lumped together as provider-patient context:

Placebos may cause placebo effects in some people in some contexts.

Now again we have spread our simple placebo causing its effects so vaguely and thinly that looking for its distinguishing features is like looking for molecules of medicine in a homeopathic remedy. We are saying only that a patient taking what appears to be a drug may get better or worse despite the apparent drug or with the help of the apparent drug or for some other reason or many reasons. Moreover these statements do not describe only placebo effects from fakery, but placebo effects from any intervention or context including drugs and surgery. The statement could be further revised to describe all interventions and contexts:

> Medical interventions may cause placebo effects in some people in some contexts.

This version forces us to consider what is special about each intervention in each context for each person being treated. To do this we need to relate placebo theory to each particular theory of the treatment in each situation. But that would be difficult to do for all varieties of disease and illness in all medical specialties.

So far the statements have not referred to the particular medical condition being treated. The next revision corrects this omission:

> Medical interventions may cause placebo effects in some people suffering from some medical conditions in some contexts.

We might formulate theories of diabetes and placebo, pain relief and placebo, Parkinson's disease and placebo, to name a few. This approach resembles the current research program that finds different placebo mechanisms for pain than for Parkinson's disease. But then we would have so many different intersecting specific treatment-condition-placebo theories that we would have to abandon hope for any coherent unified placebo theory. At that point what unified coherent work does talk of placebo do?

Placebo theory has recently become dominated by talk of expectation and conditioning. Conditioning is conceived as an unconscious process, in contrast to expectation that is deemed to be conscious. The expectation-versus-conditioning dichotomy has been described in these terms:

> There is not a single mechanism of the placebo effect and not a single placebo effect—but many. So we have to look for different mechanisms in different medical conditions and in different therapeutic interventions. Expectation and anticipation of clinical benefit play a crucial role when conscious physiological functions are involved, whereas classical conditioning takes place in unconscious physiological functions (Benedetti 2009).

Now we have questions not only internal to each construct of expectation or conditioning but also overarching questions about their relationship to each other and to placebo. Our simple descriptions of placebo can be modified to include expectation and conditioning:

> Medical interventions may cause placebo effects in some people suffering from some medical conditions in some contexts.

> Natural course of disease may account for what appear to be placebo effects.

> Expectation plays a role in conscious physiological functions.

> Conditioning takes place in unconscious physiological functions.

We have come a long way from the basic description that placebos cause placebo effects. It's no longer apparent how these statements are related. Placebo, natural course, expectation, conditioning, conscious, unconscious: what's the connection? We have enough problems understanding the conscious and the unconscious, if those terms have any traction at all in the context of physiological functions, without deeming conscious expectation and unconscious conditioning to be aspects of yet another mystery, placebo.

One approach is to weigh the respective contributions to placebo of conditioning and expectation. Stewart-Williams (2004) relegates conditioning to a minor role, arguing that, "expectancies are implicated in most placebo effects." Stewart-Williams and Podd (2004) claim to dissolve the expectancy versus conditioning debate altogether. They say that, "expectancy theory provides a partial account of the mediation of placebo effects, and conditioning procedures are one among several factors shaping such effects." Others find separate mechanisms of expectation and conditioning. Colloca and Miller (2011) suggest theorizing placebo and nocebo in terms of learning. They say that, "Learning and associated mechanisms have been demonstrated to be key mediators of expectations and placebo responses." But what is added by referring to expectation and conditioning as placebo mechanisms or grouping placebo and nocebo together as learning mediators of expectation which in turn mediates placebo responses? Leave out the notion of placebo. Then theories of expectation, conditioning and learning, or new theories that may replace them, could more directly be conceived in relation to observed treatment outcomes.

Conditioning theory has a long history in animal studies, as everyone knows from being conditioned to associate the name Pavlov with the words dog, bell and salivate. Expectation theory by contrast is based in human psychology. Learning theory itself has a vast literature encompassing numerous levels. All may have something to say about health outcomes but they are at a different level from that of neurochemistry even if they are related. Lumping these notions together as placebo leads to conceptual confusion no less than when ancient medicine gathered observations of various bodily fluids under the umbrella of humors.

Moreover, expectation and conditioning are not the only relevant factors. If the power of placebo is the power of suggestion, what are the bounds of suggestion and how does it differ from hypnosis? If suggestible people respond more to placebo treatments, what is a suggestible personality and how does suggestion influence expectation? Kirch (1999) for one expressly connects suggestion to expectancy: "response expectancy should stand as the most parsimonious explanation for hypnotic suggestibility." Again the placebo concept is shuffled off to something else, perhaps to suggestion, that in turn may be shuffled off to expectancy, or perhaps vice versa.

Expect provider expectation

An unstated assumption when talking of expectation and conditioning in placebo theory is that it's the patient's expectation and conditioning since the placebo effect is observed in the patient. Yet we should also consider the provider's expectation and conditioning and the collaboration between patient and provider.

To bring the point to the foreground from a different perspective, many researchers believe that some people respond to placebos while others do not, or at least that there is a range of responsiveness among people that is relatively stable and independent of contextual factors. So we end up with the notion of placebo responder that seems to say something about certain people. But we don't have a corresponding label for placebo effect providers who produce placebo effects in placebo responders. Yet some providers are more effective than others.

If we want to include the provider of the placebo in placebo theory, we might include the physician in clinical practice or experimenter in medical research as a kind of placebo or contextual effect, but currently we do this with a slightly different label, not as placebo effect provider but perhaps experimenter effect or white coat effect. It seems strange to refer to powerful people, who administer powerful placebos, by the color of their clothing, or say they are mere context, or consider them to be placebos, as if they are in the same category as sugar pills.

Consider instead the possibility that providers of placebos have expectations that they communicate, directly or indirectly, to patients who expect themselves to meet the expectations of their providers who also have expectations of themselves and what they must achieve in their providing capacities. In clinical practice, the placebo provider treats the patient in the expectation of improvement. Patients usually know that they are expected to improve and want to meet expectations.

In medical experiments, the provider intervenes in the lives of experimental subjects, as they expect, to improve their lives and the lives of others who may benefit from the experiment. It's not enough to say that blinding keeps experimental subjects ignorant of researchers' expectations and researchers ignorant of subjects' responses. Placebo providers communicate their expectations by providing treatments, typically with instructions that set expectations. Even if neither provider nor recipient knows what's in the treatment, nevertheless they all know the objective is to get better. Apart from infants, who does not know that they are expected to improve when treated or that the aim of medicine and medical research is to help people get better? We all know the game. Placebo and expectation are inseparable, but the notion of placebo skews the focus of inquiry onto things, the sugar pills, while diminishing the focus on the placebo providers who don't even have their own name in placebo theory.

Placebo responders please respond

Nobody knows how to identify the placebo responder. Studies that try to distinguish placebo responders from non-responders have provided equivocal results (Kaptchuk et al. 2008, Benedetti et al. 2010). The current approach is to attempt the usual biomedical reduction of observed effects to their neurochemical, genetic, psychological or other diagnostic and prognostic markers. This magic bullet approach seeks the genetic or chemical marker or personality test that shows who will respond to placebos so we could then explain and control placebos and their effects on responders.

In clinical practice, placebo responders could be identified and treated with due regard to their responsiveness. In medical research, pharmaceutical companies could use these markers to weed out placebo responders from experimental trials. Without placebo responders, their control groups wouldn't respond as well to placebos as they do now, so the experimental drugs would show relatively greater differences when compared with the carefully selected non-responder controls. With these incentives, why has the placebo responder been so elusive? It's a conceptual problem, not just a matter of more funding for more experimental research and better methodologies.

In part it's because the purported distinction between placebo responder and non-responder is a false dichotomy. The solution is not just to compromise, saying for example that there could be a continuum from no placebo response through partial response to full response. As with many other dichotomies, the responder-no-responder pair raises more questions than it answers. Given the many complex factors that could influence a person's response, how do we isolate the one factor or a few key factors that determine who responds? Of the various things that could be called responses to treatments, including not just desired positive responses but also negative responses, which things matter? Having deemed certain things to be responses that matter, how much of each of these things must be observed before it is recorded as a response? Is a placebo responder someone who always or usually responds to a particular fake treatment? Or who responds some of the time or the majority of times? Or who responds more fully than most people, and if so how full does a response need to be to make someone a responder? Or is a placebo responder someone who has a consistent response to a particular treatment when suffering various medical conditions? Or only one condition? Or a consistent response to any treatment for any condition? How does a response in an experiment relate to a response in clinical practice? These are just some of the questions that pop out when a complex network is squeezed into a pair of opposites, placebo responder and non-responder.

Those who believe placebo responders are different kinds of people from non-responders claim to know that someone is a placebo responder by observing the person's response. Two millenia ago, Galen was said to have reasoned that everyone who drinks a particular remedy recovers, so the remedy fails only when used to treat incurable cases. Incurable cases are the non-responders. Similarly, we could reason that everyone responds to placebos, except those who don't, the non-responders. This circular reasoning has been embroidered with concepts such as conditioning, expectancy and suggestibility. So for instance one could claim that there is some evidence that placebo responders are suggestible (De Pascalis et al. 2002). What, then, is it to be suggestible? Nobody really knows. We do know, however, that everyone is responsive and suggestible if we exclude those we deem not to be. The conceptual loop circles around swallowing its own tail. Better to avoid thinking in terms of placebo and placebo responders altogether.

Placebo effects without placebos

Clever open-hidden (or overt-covert) experimental methodology has created another problem for the placebo concept. With respect to knowledge of the treatment, an open-hidden experiment is the inverse of a traditional placebo-controlled experiment. In a placebo-controlled experiment, every experimental subject gets the same information about the treatment but not the same treatment. The treatment and placebo are made to look the same to fool everyone. In an open-hidden experiment, every experimental subject gets the same treatment but different information. For example, morphine appears to become a more effective analgesic when the patient is told about it than when the treatment is administered covertly (Colloca and Benedetti 2005).

The aim is to compare the effects of different knowledge and expectations rather than different substances and medical techniques: "the difference between the outcome following the overt and covert application represents the placebo (or psychological) component of the therapy, even though no placebo is given" (Benedetti et al. 2006). The placebo effect is thus extended to include instances in which placebos are either present or absent.

Can a purported cause, placebo, produce a purported effect, placebo effect, without the presence of the purported cause? Open-hidden placebo experiments are not the only examples of differences in outcomes attributed to placebos in the absence of placebos. For instance, as discussed later, adding a brand label to a bottle can influence the perception of its contents. If placebos are not necessary to generate placebo-related effects, then what is necessary? If encouraging words and brand labels are placebo-related, then what isn't placebo-related?

Expanding placebo to placebo-related grafts ever more complex epicycles on a placebo-centered universe to save the troublesome engrained placebo concept. Why bother? Open-hidden experiments provide evidence that words and environments appear to reduce suffering, in part by stimulating release of endogenous opioids. Patients who don't know what treatment they received may suffer from that very lack of knowledge while patients who are told they are getting the drug may tend to have greater expectations and report better outcomes. If there are no placebos in the experiment, why say these eperiments are placebo-related and not expectation-related, knowledge-controlled, hope-induced or some other term that expresses more directly the idea that there are no placebos?

Even these terms are lacking and retain links to the notion of placebo. Everything is related in some way, if only in that we can conceive of the things and relate them. Placebo is therefore food-related, happiness-related and history-related, to the extent that we can conceive of relations between placebo and food, happiness or history or anything else. Saying placebo-related doesn't convey much about what's happening but does expand and further entrench the domain of placebo.

Current theories of placebo include notions of conditioning and suggestion as well as expectation, so to say placebo-related implies conditioning and suggestion as well as expectation. But open-hidden experiments aim to control expectation, not to condition or hypnotize the experimental subjects. If the terminology were more specific rather than expanded to include placebo-related notions, then we would have to commit to a theory in which open-hidden experiments are based on expectation, belief, knowledge, conditioning, learning or something else, but not a generalized notion of placebo-relatedness.

Moreover, conflicting views appear among those who call for a broadened notion of placebo-related effects that occur without placebos. Benedetti (2008) argues that "the term placebo effect is too restrictive and should be extended to related phenomena that share similar mechanisms." But in an earlier paper Benedetti and colleagues wrote that placebo terminology should be limited not extended:

...it might be time to limit the use of the term placebo effect to those situations in which inert (dummy) medical treatments are given ... However, it is worth noting that even if a placebo is given, there is no such thing as a placebo effect, since this term deflects our gaze from what is really important (the meaning and the meaning-induced expectations) and aims it at what is not (the inert pills and, in general, the inert medical treatments) (Benedetti et al. 2003).

Conflicting attempts by great minds to capture the placebo notion are evidence that the great effort required to preserve placebo might be better devoted elsewhere. Their struggle to carve out a consistent, comprehensive class of things that include placebo effects and placebo-related effects is futile in the same way that it was futile to try to carve out a consistent, comprehensive class of medical things called humors. These examples suggest at least the following conflicting options:

—Limit placebo effects to observations that follow fake medical treatments in controlled experiments.
—Include observations that follow fake medical treatments in uncontrolled clinical practice.
—Extend placebo effects to include observations in the absence of fake treatments.
—Acknowledge the confusion inherent in the notion of placebo but keep saying placebo in any event while waiting for something better.
—Stop saying placebo and placebo effects.

Only the last of these options will avoid the problems of placebo now and prepare the path to medicine after placebo.

7 Placebo Science

The current placebo paradigm is a creature of medical and scientific methods. There is no general agreement, however, about methods in science or in medicine. Arguments rage over how science actually works, including whether science is strictly speaking rational and logical, how social factors influence scientific reasoning and many other fundamental questions. What, for example, is the proper way to infer general principles about placebo based on observations of individual cases? Consider the following accounts of reasoning at various stages of medical and scientific methodologies. These are not the only variations; for instance Bayesian methods of inference are omitted, but the following should be sufficient.

An inductive account of science asserts that scientists infer general laws from specific empirical observations. A common example used to illustrate induction is the observation that the sun has appeared at the horizon every morning in the past and therefore we can infer and predict that as a rule the sun will rise every day in future. The prediction resulting from the rule or hypothesis is testable. We can conduct a test every morning at sunrise.

Unlike deduction, induction needs more information than is contained in the premises. The additional information, the evidential basis for the argument, is subject to the uncertainties of the world. In the example of the rising sun, one uncertainty is whether a collision with another object might alter the movement of our planet such that the sun no longer appears to rise. When reasoning by induction, a cluster of concepts applies including confidence, uncertainty, probability, effect size, incidence rate, exposure, and risk rather than perfect certainty.

All of these are relevant to the relations between medical evidence and the notion of placebo. An inductive account of placebo might go like this: improvements have regularly been observed in some patients treated with fake drugs and procedures. For example, Beecher observed a powerful analgesic effect in severely wounded soldiers injected with water instead of morphine. He found the effect regularly occurring in 35% of patients in a variety of conditions. Therefore fake drugs and procedures, let's call them dummies or placebos, and their observed effects, let's call them placebo effects, are connected by the general principle or law in medicine that can be inferred from these observations, namely that placebos cause placebo effects. Observation shows that the sun rises each day, and by similar reasoning observation shows that approximately one third of patients exhibit placebo effects.

This inductive account of placebo doesn't fit comfortably with the sunrise effect, however. Scientists do not generate rules about the Sun in that way, nor do they speak of the sunrise effect in the way that many people speak of the placebo effect. There is no mysterious sunrise effect. Sunrise has been explained by astronomers and physicists while placebo has no agreed explanation. If placebos always relieved pain, or if placebo effects were modeled by tractable mathematical expressions as are the movements of the Sun and Earth, that explain why placebos usually have no effect while the sun rises on more than 35% of mornings, these accounts could be somewhat more alike. But that is not our world.

A different view is of science as a closed deductive (or hypothetical-deductive or hypothetical-predictive) system. Under a deductive view, scientists begin with general premises from which, if they don't make any errors, they deduce inevitable, logically unassailable conclusions. In medicine, for instance, an observer starts with some hypothesis that explains what is observed of the patient, then tests the hypothesis. If you believe that medicine is such a logically tidy science, then what is wrong with the following reasoning?

Improvements in patients who receive inert treatments are placebo effects.

I observed improvements in patients who received inert treatment.

Therefore I observed placebo effects.

This is merely a circular exercise of defining placebo effects in terms of inert treatments, but explains nothing about what is going on given the many possible explanations for the observations. Instead, the logical conclusion could be stated as a prediction. For instance:

If a patient is told that the placebo is a powerful drug, then the patient will show a placebo effect.

This is just another definition of placebo effect. It is like saying: if a patient takes a sleeping pill, the patient will show a sleep effect. Such circular reasoning is reminiscent of Molière's famous virtus dormitiva or dormitive principle that satirically explains the soporific effect of opium merely by assigning a Latin label. Consider related reasoning stated in conditional form:

If there are observed placebo effects then the treatment is a placebo.

I did not observe placebo effects.

Therefore the treatment was not a placebo.

Again this is a definitional exercise disguised as empirical research based on observation and falsification. What does it mean not to observe placebo effects? Is it what the observer decides was not observed? Was anything else happening that might interfere with a placebo effect? Perhaps the logic would be improved if we specified that placebo effects are non-specific effects:

Placebo effects, as opposed to effects of real drugs and procedures, are non-specific effects.

I observed non-specific effects in patients after placebo treatment.

Therefore I observed placebo effects.

This chain of thought depends on there being readily distinguishable non-specific effects and on non-specific effects being the product of placebo treatments and nothing else. What exactly would be a reliable observation of a non-specific effect? We would not be much better off if the statements referred to context effects or meaning responses. Perhaps a return to Beecher would help:

If Beecher is correct, I will observe improvement in 35% of patients treated with placebos.

I observed improvement in 35% of patients treated with placebos.

Therefore Beecher is correct: the placebo effect is powerful.

Replicating Beecher's findings is suggestive of further investigation but not conclusive. Although the matching observation of 35% appears to support a general law, this example merely provides a deductive frame around an inductive or abductive account. Many factors other than placebo could explain the observations and Beecher's theory is not the only one that fits.

Consider also the logic of clinical trials that compare treatments. A trial that compares an experimental treatment with placebo goes something like this when the experimental treatment is deemed to work:

I observed a significantly better outcome in the experimental group than in the placebo group.

Therefore the experimental treatment works better than placebo.

This result does not say much about placebo, which remains an unexplained black box comparator. The example leaves out the following premise:

If patients have significantly better outcomes in the experimental group, then the experimental treatment works better than placebo.

Of course this group comparison rule is not a general rule that applies to anyone outside the experiment or to any individual patient. For an experiment that does not demonstrate a difference between groups:

If there is no significant difference between treatment and placebo groups, the experimental treatment does not work better than placebo.

I observed an insignificant difference in outcome between groups.

Therefore the experimental treatment does not work better than placebo.

Now this conclusion does not tell us much about either the experimental treatment or placebo. How close were the two groups? How sensitive is the test? Why was the difference between the groups deemed to be insignificant? What explains the results? The experiment does not show that the treatments have the same effects, but only that no observable difference appeared in the particular experiment.

For those relatively uncommon clinical trials with both a placebo group and a no-treatment group, the reasoning broadly appears to be something like this:

The outcome in the placebo group was (the same, better, worse) than in the no-treatment group.

Therefore placebo is (the same as, no worse than, more powerful than, less powerful than) no treatment.

Here placebo remains a black box that in some cases correlates with different outcomes than no treatment does. Among other issues, we are also faced with the problem of distinguishing between placebo and no treatment, and in particular accounting for the expectations of people in a no-treatment group. More generally, it's not clear that the reasoning behind clinical trials is strictly deductive rather than taking another path, perhaps among the following examples.

Other accounts of science include the theory of null hypothesis testing, promoted by Ronald A. Fisher, that focused on two possible outcomes, rejection of the null hypothesis or no conclusion. Fisher's theory of reasoning about experiments can be conceived in terms of the general non-inductive theory of falsification, which is often associated with Karl Popper, who rejected induction as the basis of scientific reasoning.

It is difficult to conceive of an experiment that could falsify the circular definition of placebo as something that causes placebo effects, or non-specific effects or context effects. Fisher's null hypothesis testing is also unappealing to many, particularly those who pay for expensive medical experiments and want a clear positive conclusion for their money rather than a finding of no conclusion. Experimenters in medicine rarely stick to purely Fisherian methods, often preferring a combination of approaches due to Fisher as modified by Jerzy Neyman and Egon Pearson.

Neyman-Pearson methodology aims to find rules for deciding among alternatives rather than interpreting statistical evidence as justification for beliefs. A quintessential case for decision rules is in quality control. For instance, the manufacturer of a medical device needs to test and reject dangerous defective devices before they are delivered to patients. No testing or measuring process is without error, however. If a device is tested repeatedly the results will nevertheless not be the same each time. Tolerances for acceptance and rejection must be selected to protect patients by ensuring that inevitable errors will result in rejection of a safe device rather than delivery of a defective device. To err on the safe side implies that there is good reason to believe that some safe devices will be rejected as if they were defective. But to accept or reject a given device does not require any particular belief, only the action of accepting or rejecting according to some specific tolerance.

The same reasoning can be applied to any choice among hypotheses, without commitment to believing any hypothesis. We could deem an observation to be a placebo effect or not based on some acceptance tolerance without commitment to any hypothesis. We would nevertheless need some basis for our accepted tolerance limit and in any event that would leave us without a placebo theory.

The goal of making choices also appears in other views of science. Two related alternatives are inference to the best explanation and abduction (a term usually credited to C.S. Pierce). There is some disagreement about these terms, with some theoreticians equating them and others finding large distinctions (for instance Campos 2011). An example of abduction in medical diagnosis is the following data combined with selected plausible explanation and inference (adapted from Upshur 1997):

I observe that these children have fevers (data).

Most children with fevers have viral infections (selected plausible explanation among others).

These children probably have a viral infection (inference).

The observation of fevers raises the probability that it's a viral infection. In other circumstances, for instance during an epidemic of non-viral origin, a different plausible hypothesis with different probabilities may result in a different inference despite similar data. Abductive reasoning about placebo might go like this:

A surprising effect is observed: that patients given sugar pills report less pain.

But if placebos were powerful, then the effect would be no surprise.

So there is reason to believe that placebos are powerful.

Despite the surface form of this reasoning, we are left cycling around in a conceptual circle without greater understanding of what is going on behind the placebo terminology.

A common general example of judgment required to choose among competing explanations is curve fitting. Given scattered data points on a graph, countless possible lines can be drawn to abstract or generalize the ideal function that expresses the relationship among the points. The observer (in medicine perhaps the physician, epidemiologist or biostatistician) selects the theoretical curve that best fits the data. As Toulmin (1961) has pointed out, however, by analogy to the evolution of biological species, not all conceivable theories could survive the competition with other theories:

> ...philosophers sometimes assert that a finite set of empirical observations can always be explained in terms of an infinite number of hypotheses. The basis for this remark is the simple observation that through any finite set of points an infinite number of mathematical curves can be constructed. If there were no more to 'explanation' than curve-fitting, this doctrine would have some bearing on scientific practice. In fact, the scientist's problem is very different: in an intellectual situation which presents a variety of demands, his task is—typically—to accommodate some new discovery to his inherited ideas, without needlessly jeopardizing the intellectual gains of his predecessors. This kind of problem has an order of complexity quite different from that of simple curve-fitting: far from his having an infinite number of possibilities to choose between, it may be a stroke of genius for him to imagine even a single one. The scientist might, in fact, retort to the logician as the French painter Courbet is said to have replied to the art-critics by commenting that 'it is a hard enough matter to paint a picture at all, let alone a good picture'.

There is an uncertainty and provisional nature associated with data. Given more data, what is considered to be the best fit today may change tomorrow; such inference is always provisional. This is not to say there are no certainties. Death and taxes, as they say, are certain. But experts are rarely asked to opine about certainties.

Their expertise is most valuable when they make the best decision, or in this context when they infer the best explanation, under uncertainty. In medicine there is no shortage of uncertainty. It is uncertain where placebo theory and data cross paths, but it is likely that the current placebo curve is not the best or most plausible fit.

Even if questions about placebo science were answered, unresolved issues would remain about the extent to which medicine is a science or uses scientific methods. Scientific reasoning, whether inductive, deductive, abductive or some other form, may apply only in part or not at all to medical reasoning.

Expert views expressed on the connections between science and medicine are all over the map. Surgeon William Inlow (1946) says medicine is a science, art, professional practice and social relationship, a whole in its own right. Science writer Bernard Dixon (1978) says medicine, offering both comfort and cure, is not synonymous with science. Virologist Michael Stoker (1980) begins an article with the reductionist axiom, "Medicine, as we all know, is one of the branches of biology." Medical philosophers Edmund Pellegrino and David Thomasma (1981) say medicine is science, art and virtue. Internist Eric Cassell (2004) says medicine is neither art nor science. Philosopher Miriam Solomon (2008) refuses to cut the subject in half, arguing instead that the dichotomy between art and science of medicine is not helpful. Kathryn Montgomery (2006), professor of medical humanities, says physicians pretend to be scientists while working quite differently. Biostatistician Barker Bausell (2007) says medicine is applied science. Medical historian Jaclyn Duffin (2010) says medicine is not a science but an applied technology or an art that makes extensive use of science. In Delkeskamp-Hayes and Cutter (1993) seventeen authors consider, without reaching a consensus, whether medicine is science, technology or art. Within this divergence of opinion we find a divergence of roles for placebo in medical science, art, craft or some other division.

Then where does placebo logically fit? Should the collected observations of unexplained improvement be assigned to the placebo category? For those who reject an inductive account of medicine, does a falsification model apply? How would placebo theory be falsified? To the extent that the methods of science are debated, the application of science to medicine is contested, and the placebo notion is unclear, placebo inference is also not clear.

Placebo as confirmation bias

The placebo construct is not ordinarily viewed as a consequence of bias in human reasoning. Indeed, far from being an example of bias, placebo appears not only to be compatible with the norms of good reasoning but also is seen as the enemy of bias in clinical trials where placebo controls are intended to eliminate biases. But what if the notion of placebo itself is the consequence of confirmation bias, the tendency to confirm rather than challenge one's own opinions? If we believe in the power of placebo, then we are likely to accept supporting evidence and criticize other evidence. If we believe that homeopathy cannot cure cancer, we will be skeptical of reports that homeopathy does cure cancer, choosing what we claim to know and believe over the possibility of miracles. If we believe in the power of homeopathy, we will find that power exists. Indeed such bias could be viewed as the consequence of holding any theory instead of an opposing theory.

Merely asking the question "Is this a placebo effect?" could make finding a placebo effect more likely. Asking whether placebo is a category in the world also focuses attention on that category and suggests a positive answer to the question. When looking at the history of medicine, throughout which almost any intervention has been said to work, it's easy to infer that there is a special power in any medical intervention, namely placebo power. When observing, as Beecher and many others since have done, that apparently ineffective treatments paradoxically relieve pain almost as well as powerful analgesics, then it makes sense to look for other examples of paradoxical successes. Few people would see examples that refute the placebo hypothesis, if indeed such a thing were possible to observe. It's hard to see pain relief after a water injection as anything but confirmation of a placebo hypothesis. As you look at the world through a placebo lens, you will surely find placebos and placebo effects.

A widely cited review by psychologist Raymond Nickerson (1998), selected from a voluminous literature, considers bias in various fields including medicine; he argues that confirmation bias appears in so many guises that it ranks as the single leading error in human reasoning. He also blames confirmation bias for many other phenomena including persistence of unfounded beliefs and outdated scientific theories. From Nickerson's account, it could be said that rather than being one of many perceptual and reasoning problems, confirmation bias is the mother of all biases. Nickerson points out that instances said to confirm a hypothesis are often illusory. They are confirmatory in a psychological sense but not in a logical sense. So for instance finding many stories of patients who suffer less pain after placebo treatment might appear to confirm the hypothesis that powerful placebo effects exist. But those positive instances must logically be contrasted with stories of patients who did not improve after placebo treatment, the large majority, together with stories of what happened to patients who received no treatment at all. That most patients do not appear to benefit from Beecher's powerful placebo effect has had remarkably little logical effect on placebo theory.

Consider again the story of Mr Wright whose tumors apparently melted after placebo treatment. His story appears to confirm a placebo hypothesis. But the confirmation is illusory. We would need to look at cases that did not improve and at cases that did not have placebo intervention. That is, Mr Wright's story is only one type among at least four types that must be considered: placebo with improvement, placebo without improvement, improvement without placebo, or no placebo and no improvement. To say Mr Wright or any story of placebo improvement matters is to say only that confirming stories matter. That may be psychologically satisfying but what matters logically are the disconfirming stories in addition to the confirming ones.

As Nickerson points out, perhaps his habit of seeing confirmation bias everywhere is an example of his own confirmation bias. Perhaps the argument here for not seeing and not saying placebo is another example of confirmation bias. That is an unavoidable possibility. Will the unbiased person please raise your hand?

Unspecified placebo

To talk of placebo does not require any medical specialty: we don't say cardiological placebo or gastroeneterological placebo. Placebo can be involved in almost any treatment for any condition, and its extension to placebo-related things in the absence of placebos boldly takes the concept where no medical concept has gone before. Placebo is not even limited by time or place. Or put in the negative, nothing in medicine or almost nothing is not a placebo. Medicine itself by contrast has become subdivided into multiple specialties and subspecialties. Even general medical practice has become a medical specialty.

The all-inclusiveness of placebo plagues the broad range of underlying placebo ontology that includes various substances, bodily systems and multiple levels of analysis. Given the convenient class named placebo, we are tempted to fill it with examples of placebo things. The class becomes a catch-all for mysterious effects and their mechanisms. According to Shapiro and Shapiro (1997) placebo can be:

—any treatment (including drugs, surgery, psychotherapy and
   quack therapy)
—whether inert or active
—no matter how potentially specific
—for any symptom or disease
—no matter who administers the placebo
—in any manner (oral, parenteral, topical, magical)
—through all of medical history
—in all societies and cultures

Placebo transcends all boundaries while other aspects of medicine
are bounded by something, whether it is time, location, system,
method or something else. The human body in biomedicine is
conceived in terms of bodily systems and organs, and experts who
study the body are divided by specialty. Brain tissue inhabits a
different conceptual space than blood, each occupying their own
separate disciplines, journals and departments. Placebo, however,
is not bounded by disease, symptom, origin, anatomy, organ, system
or any other boundary that delimits placebo as a particular class of
things.

Many other terms cross boundaries. For example, surgeons
remove tissue. Analgesics remove pain. Dentists remove teeth.
These could be considered to be instances of removals. Removal
effects are the category of effects caused by removals, whether the
removal be limbs, teeth, headaches, worries or anything else
removed. Such a broad notion of removal effects, however, does
not fill an emptiness in medical theory. Conversely a generic term
such as additions could be used for added tissue, skin grafts, blood
transfusions, dental implants, added value and anything else added
rather than removed. Like the manufactured notions of removal
effects and addition effects, placebo effects are less useful
groupings than meet the eye.

8 Desperately Seeking Meaning

Returning now to proposed alternatives to placebo language, consider the shift from placebo to meaning and context. Eric Cassell (2004), for instance, puts meaning at the center of his view of suffering. His thesis is that:

> Meanings are essential to everything that persons do... in persons meaning is the medium through which thought flows into the body and the body flows into thought... Meaning is not merely an epiphenomenon—it provides direct access to the sick or well person's body.

Howard Brody (1987) offers a story-telling, narrative approach in which what is a meaningful stimulus of a placebo response is integrated by the story of the particular patient:

> A story that makes sense, implies enhanced social support and caring, and tends to lead toward mastery and control of the illness will maximize the perceived (and objective) relief of the sickness episode: a story that promotes meaninglessness, social isolation, and helplessness will do the opposite.

Howard Spiro (1986) takes a view that is consistent with Brody, Cassell and other meaning theorists:

> I take the response to a placebo as a testament to our common humanity, to most peoples' need for community and a friend in time of troubles. Most men and women are not lone wolves.

Daniel Moerman (2002a, 2002b, 2003) has been a prominent advocate for language change in relation to placebo. He too would like to see the term placebo effect banished from medical terminology. In its place he would use the term meaning response which he says are the physiological or psychological effects of meaning in the treatment of illness. The meaning response, however, is deeply connected to the placebo notion: "the placebo effect in the strict sense is only a special case of the meaning response" (2002b). A related proposal is to use the terms response and effect interchangeably (Benedetti 2009).

In the context of clinical trials, Moerman (2003) says the meaning response is "a residual increment of improvement" in the control group and is the same as the "true placebo effect", what remains after accounting for natural history, bias, regression to the mean and other sources of perceived placebo effect. Moerman's meaning response is not limited to the control group or to experiments but is a general description of responses to treatment. The meaning response has been criticized, however, as vague and a catch-all for unaccounted effects (Thompson et al. 2009).

Meaning proponents have contributed valuable new ways of thinking. Yet they and others have not managed to break free from some of the problems of placebo. Meaning response retains the one-handed dispositional language of placebo effect, conceived passively in terms of response, as placebo is conceived in terms of effect. It's also unclear how meaning is related to expectation and conditioning. Moerman prefers meaning to expectation because meaning responses do not always involve expectation. By contrast, pain expert Patrick Wall (1996) says meaning actually is a name for expectation: "Expectation is given a number of related names, such as belief, faith, confidence, enthusiasm, response bias, meaning, credibility, transference, anticipation…"

Attempts have been made to measure meaning. More than half a century ago, while Beecher (1955) was promoting the powerful placebo, Osgood et al. (1957) set out to develop a quantitative measure of meaning in psychology, just as psychologists have developed measures of intelligence, affect and other difficult concepts. With the benefit of early computer technology, Osgood and colleagues created a technique for measuring meaning that they termed the semantic differential. Experimental subjects rated concepts in terms of adjectives presented as opposites along a seven-point scale. For example, a concept could be rated along scales of good or bad and active or passive. Data collected in this manner was factored and conceptualized as a spatial matrix relating concepts to the scaled polar opposites.

Is this the same meaning as that of medical meaning theorists? Osgood and colleagues observe that there as many meanings of the word meaning as there are disciplines dealing with language. These include linguistic, psychological, representational and relational interpretations. They also acknowledge the criticism that they were measuring emotive reactions to words, or correlations between word stimuli and linguistic responses, not meaning. They agree that they too use the word meaning in several senses: "whether or not it is *meaning* that we are measuring, then, would seem to be merely a matter of choice of terms." Despite this fundamental ambiguity, the semantic differential, like its contemporary, Beecher's powerful placebo effect, has since evolved into a staple of current research.

Even if meaning response could be discerned and measured, its many meanings would still have to be disambiguated. And to replace placebo theory with meaning theory is to retain much of what is troubling about placebo without gaining enough in return for the effort.

Demanding the context for context effects

The term context has become central to placebo theory and indeed placebo effects have been called effects of therapeutic context or context effects (Di Blasi et al. 2001). Behavioral researchers have a similar category that they call the demand characteristics of an experiment (Rosnow and Rosenthal 1997). As an example of the influence of experimental context, Martin Orne (1962) writes:

> Just about any request which could conceivably be asked of the subject by a reputable investigator is legitimized by the quasi-magical phrase, "This is an experiment," and the shared assumption that a legitimate purpose will be served by the subject's behavior. A somewhat trivial example of this legitimization of requests is as follows: A number of casual acquaintances were asked whether they would do the experimenter a favor; on their acquiescence, they were asked to perform five push-ups. Their response tended to be amazement, incredulity and the question "Why?" Another similar group of individuals were asked whether they would take part in an experiment of brief duration. When they agreed to do so, they too were asked to perform five push-ups. Their typical response was "Where?"

Context effects are not limited to experiments, however. Context effects have been given a broad scope. They are described as the non-specific effects, that which isn't specific to the biomedical contents of treatment, and are attributed to all sorts of influences, including relationships, words, emotions and perceptions in a medical context. Context is reminiscent of Jorge Luis Borges' fictional classification of animals that includes embalmed ones and mermaids. All treatments are administered in some context so there must be something more to the broad contextual conception of placebo than a vague connection to context.

One could imagine a spectrum of conditions, and responses to treatments for those conditions, perhaps along an artificial line distinguishing functional from organic injury. One might anticipate that the subtleties of treatments for chronic unexplained back pain depend more on psychosocial context than do emergency treatments for penetrating gunshot wounds. Invisible chronic pain seems more contextual and subjective than visible traumatic injuries. But such acute injuries are the very examples from battlefield experiences that inspired Beecher's seminal investigations of what he called the powerful placebo effect.

Context effect, non-specific effect, meaning response and similar replacements for placebo are no less mysterious than placebo. Whatever their subtle differences, these terms are alike enough to be considered to be synonyms (Di Blasi et al. 2001, Koshi and Short 2007). They are black boxes within black boxes.

Switching paradigms: the performance effect

The placebo effect resembles a performance or audience effect. Imagine that you are a stranger visiting this world, unfamiliar with human ways. You happen upon a small crowd watching a man dressed in black. As you study the faces in the audience, suddenly and for no apparent reason they burst into smiles and laughter. Then they quietly watch again. Then more laughter. Then quiet. This cycle of attention then explosive reaction then attention happens several times.

Watching closely, you see that the man manipulates small objects. Playing cards. Coins. A rabbit. A hat. He talks constantly. From your viewpoint standing behind him, what he does is obvious. He merely hides a coin in the palm of his hand. The audience reacts. To be exact, not everybody gasps or laughs equally loudly or frequently. Some members of the audience could be deemed to be performance responders who are particularly influenced by the performance effect.

To someone who does not understand the meaning of the magician's words and actions the performance effect is mysterious. Viewed only mechanistically, the crowd gasps and claps for no apparent reason. Why does showing them the ace of hearts create a performance effect? Why do they fail to react to the ace of spades? The initial hypothesis that the ace of hearts has special powers turns out to be false. The ace of hearts was selected by someone in the audience then replaced in the deck. They expected the ace of hearts to be somewhere in the shuffled deck, so they laughed when the magician appeared to extract that very card from the ear of a child in the audience.

What do we gain from constructing the notion of a performance or audience effect? Nothing, and much of what is happening is obscured by such terminology and related notions such as performance or audience responders. Similarly the physician-magician with a magic inert pill seems to induce a mysterious placebo effect in the patient-audience. On a different conception of the patient, however, the patient is not a mechanism. The patient is a conscious person who takes meaning from the whole sickness story, with its familiar plot including diagnosis, prognosis, treatment and rehabilitation and its emotions associated with worry, pain, suffering, uncertainty, concern and reassurance. From this viewpoint, there is no surprise that, beyond drugs and other ingredients, many factors including words, rituals, colors, shapes and costs have meaningful effects.

The mechanisms may vary, as do the magician's tricks. The professional entertainer may not know for certain why some jokes and illusions get better responses than others. Full knowledge of the exact mechanism is not required to make the audience react or to improve the patient's health. But being able to observe effects does not mean there is a general class of mechanisms attributable to performances or placebos that will generate or explain either phenomenon. Neither performances nor placebos have been fully explained, yet placebo has been isolated as a special effect.

Placebo carries baggage of mystery, magic, deception, fakery, quackery and other negative connotations. Yet put positively, everything has a potential meaning. The person's interpretation of events has medical and health consequences. Any pills or syringes, including those that deliver only sugar or water, have meaning to some people. And the bigger the pill, the more expensive, the more power they are meant to contain. The big name performer and the big pill may each have big effects.

We could debate whether the performance effect would be better expressed if we were to call it the audience effect, or perhaps they should both be replaced by the phrase performing context effects. The idea that the term placebo effects could be replaced by some other term assumes that the concept of placebo and its effects is something worth preserving.

Metaphorical placebo

In a conceptual analysis of the placebo construct, psychologists Joseph Critelli and Carl Neumann (1984) considered two common placebo metaphors:

> Two dominant placebo metaphors have appeared in the literature: (a) placebos as inert rather than active ingredients and (b) placebos as nonspecific rather than specific agents. Although particularly problematic in recent years, it is important to note that placebo terminology within both metaphors has always constituted a web of overextended generalizations and internal contradictions.

These are only two of the many metaphors associated with placebo. Placebo as therapeutic context. Placebo as magic. Placebo as universal medicine. Placebo as performance. Placebo as deception. Placebo as suggestion. Placebo as expectation. Placebo as conditioning. Placebo as learning. Placebo as remembering. The broadly construed notion of placebo derives illusory support from metaphors that, as Critelli and Neumann indicate, are bound up with problematic terminology.

Paradigms, like other metaphors, attempt to shape the confusion of the world into something manageable. The current view of placebo is a metaphorical construct within a biomedical paradigm at the boundary of other metaphors, images and views. As long as we remain within the current paradigm, and accept the placebo notion in medical research and clinical practice, we don't have to think about troubling issues such as how the paradigm came to be framed as it is and whether it makes sense compared to different metaphors. Instead we can proceed to solve the puzzles, such as untangling the brain mechanisms of placebo, shared among the community of researchers who adopt the paradigm.

Purported mechanisms, concepts and ideas associated with the placebo effect have been gathered in yet another metaphor, a melting pot:

> In other words, different processes may be at work in the patient's brain in different conditions. Sometimes it is anxiety that is modulated, at some other times reward mechanisms are involved, and in some other circumstances different types of learning, or even genetic variants, may take place in placebo responsiveness. In this sense, the placebo effect is a melting pot of neuroscientific concepts and ideas, ranging from anxiety and reward mechanisms to Pavlovian conditioning and social learning, and from neurogenetics and neurophysiology to clinical practice and neuroethics (Benedetti et al. 2010).

The melting pot metaphor is an apt one for the unconstrained notion of placebo effect that mixes all medical treatments for all conditions. But if the placebo effect is a melting pot of concepts and ideas, what does that tell us about the need for the concept of placebo or its effects? Nothing specific and much that is unnecessarily confusing.

Nocebo

The concept of a negative placebo, or nocebo, shares the conceptual problems of placebo. Nocebo phenomena are said to be opposite to placebo phenomena. But what exactly does that mean? Just as placebo is an elusive concept, variously described and used, it's no surprise that the nocebo concept cannot be captured without extensive negotiation of terms. Like placebo, nocebo cannot be pinned down to inert substances or fake procedures, but appears to encompass any negative outcome in a negative context that isn't otherwise explained according to the biomedical paradigm, and so is therefore attributed to a vague notion of negative psychosocial context.

As with placebo, the dark nocebo side is supported by dramatic anecdotes such as reports of voodoo death. A powerful nocebo anecdote told in various forms is that of the priest who administered last rites to the patient in the bed next to the dying patient. That patient who received the last rites died within 15 minutes while the patient who was expected to die lived another 4 days (Spiegel 1997). As interesting as these stories are, they explain nothing about placebo or nocebo, and can be told without these mysterious notions.

Nocebo, like placebo, has been described in terms of objective reality and the power of suggestion, as in the "real nocebo procedure" of administering an inert substance with verbal suggestions (Benedetti 2009). According to Spiegel (1997) nocebo is the power of suggestibility, a conception that imports all the problems of explaining hypnosis and suggestion. The reality of nocebo, like that of placebo, is bolstered by evidence of brain activity from neuroimaging and pharmacology studies that imply both phenomena use related brain mechanisms. Mirroring the notion of placebo-related effects in the absence of inert substances, some aspects of nocebo are described as nocebo-like phenomena or nocebo-related effects (Benedetti 2009).

Yet again it's not clear how all of these things are meaningfully joined in a coherent theory. Voodoo death is often cited as a nocebo effect, but the rare voodoo example is a long way, conceptually and culturally, from experiments in which decaffeinated coffee is followed by a headache, and from the common occurrence in clinical practice of nausea in anticipation of treatment. Anticipated nausea has also been termed a conditioned nocebo effect or response (Benedetti 2009). Why is it not simply a conditioned response? Leave out the notional nocebo intermediary.

Side effects from placebo are not singularly or coherently negative since they are associated with positive belief that the treatment works. Nocebo is associated with positive belief that the treatment harms. If nocebo were truly an opposite of placebo, then more researchers would be talking about side effects of nocebo, that is, unintended positive effects of believing that a treatment harms, or paradoxical placebo and nocebo effects that are opposite to their respective positive and negative characterizations.

Even if there were no such concept as a negative placebo, placebos would still by definition be associated with some negative concepts and negative effects on patients. For instance, Miller and Kaptchuk (2008a) point out the negative values conveyed by defining placebo in terms such as inert, inactive, non-specific, dummy, sham, noise and bias. They say that placebo itself is defined by what it is not rather than by what it is. To say non-specific is to assume that specific is positive, somehow better than not being specific. Then if nocebo is the opposite of placebo, is nocebo defined by what it is rather than what it is not? Sorting out these abundant and overlapping negatives is not for the faint of heart.

At a broader level are the values implicit when placing something on one side or the other of the placebo-nocebo dichotomy. For instance, perhaps the opportunity cost of using placebo treatment when better treatment could be used is an example of a conceptual nocebo. Or for a less conceptual and very specific example, when used initially for opening blood vessels, the drug sildenafil was a failure, but when used for its unexpected side effects, and marketed as Viagra, it reached a climax for its makers and users.

Concepts of positive and negative, good and bad, help and harm, treatment effect and side effect are problematic dichotomies that infect the notion of nocebo as much as its purported placebo opposite. Again we should be wary of false dichotomies. It doesn't matter whether nocebo is just the evil twin of placebo. Neither twin is particularly useful.

Placebo evolution

The widespread observation of apparent placebo effects throughout history and across cultures has prompted many investigators to look for an evolutionary explanation. Shapiro and Shapiro (1997) conclude their overview of the history of the placebo with this question:

> Does the ubiquity of the placebo effect throughout history suggest the possibility, popular but hardly testable today, or perhaps ever, that positive placebo effects are an inherited adaptive characteristic, conferring evolutionary advantages by reducing despondency, depression, and hopelessness, and that allowed more people with the placebo trait to survive than those without it?

Evolutionary just-so stories of placebo are unlike explanations in the basic sciences. Physics and chemistry seek generalities. But evolved creatures are contingencies not generalities. Humans are the way we are because of our evolutionary history. Although humans are subject to the generalities of basic sciences, such as electromagnetic forces and the chemical properties of water, we are not predicted by them, nor is the existence of our species necessary to validate any general law.

Is the placebo predicted by or essential for any theory of evolution? Or could humans have evolved without what are now called placebo effects or responses? Did we evolve to trust doctors? The following view suggests that trust in medical authority has survival advantages:

> From an evolutionary perspective, it is tempting to speculate that social stimuli may have drug-like therapeutic properties because this is advantageous for a member of a social group. If you trust an authoritative member of your social group, be he a modern doctor or a primitive shaman, you have better chances to survive and to improve your quality of life. This "endogenous pharmacy" is made up of biochemical pathways described throughout this review that are activated by various social stimuli. Although this evolutionary perspective is only speculative, these issues are worthy of further scrutiny, as they seem likely to lead to fundamental insights into both human biology and therapeutics (Benedetti 2008).

On the contrary, evidence-based medicine explicitly deprecates trust in medical expertise and authority in preference for evidence from randomized controlled trials and systematic reviews of those trials. Evidence-based practitioners have been urged to search and trust the research literature rather than the pronouncements of expert authorities (Nunn 2008). From an evidence-based viewpoint, trust in medical authority is said to be maladaptive.

Psychologist Nicholas Humphrey (2002) draws an analogy between the body's self-repairing capability and the National Health Service. He considers the placebo to be an emergent property of the body's own managed health care system. Inspired by Humphrey, Dylan Evans (2003, 2005) also adopts the resource management metaphor, although he differs in the details. For instance, Evans says placebos inhibit the innate immune response. This inhibition view is opposite to that of Humphrey who sees the placebo as something that releases resources. A common thread in these accounts is a model of optimizing limited resources. Every organism must continually solve the problem of what to do next and with what combination of resources. But nothing is gained by giving resource allocation the name placebo.

Placebo means more than medicine

Meaning, context, expectation, belief, hope and other factors associated with placebo are not unique to medical research and clinical practice. They are general aspects of being human and indeed, placebo has been extended beyond medicine to include psychology. Jopling (2008), for instance, has suggested that the concept of psychodynamic placebos might make sense so we should design studies to investigate them. Pollo et al. (2011) have extended their conception of placebo effects to "the consequence of a general interaction between an organism and its environment." Outside of medicine and other therapeutic activities, the notion of placebo pervades popular and scientific literature where, for instance, it is common to call a deceptive influence a mere placebo. It has become difficult to find a human activity that is not to some degree tainted by placebo talk.

Consider the context of sport. When a coach urges an athlete to keep going, to try harder, we don't generally refer to any resulting performance improvement in terms of placebo effects. We call it coaching not placebo-ing. Yet just as placebo somehow appears to recruit outside contextual help in a medical context to spur the body's own pain-killing biochemicals among other effects, so the coaching context spurs the athlete's mind and body to overcome pain, run faster, jump higher, hit harder, throw farther and win. Many athletes believe they experience placebo effects (Beedie 2007). Many might also say that sporting events cause nocebo effects, such as anxiety and vomiting before competition, or injury during the event and depression after a loss.

At a more literal level of comparison between placebos in medicine and in sport, dummy substances have been ingested and injected in sporting contexts with many parallels to medical contexts. For instance, Kalasountas et al. (2007) claim that placebos help college students to lift weights while Benedetti et al. (2007) consider whether placebo use in sport is cheating. Placebo in sport may seem to be a natural extension from placebo in medicine, as medicine extends its domain from sickness to health. At times we use something external (such as coaching or water injection) to make us do something internal (run fast, feel better). But to call it placebo-ing does not add anything to our understanding of coaching or sport medicine.

Consider now the context of advertising and marketing. When people choose a product because they recognize the brand name, we don't usually call that a placebo effect. Nor do we use the term placebo-controlled trial when a product advertiser stages a taste test between a competitor's product and what the advertiser wants us to believe is the better product. Yet the brand name induces the purchaser to believe that the product is better and purchasers indeed will say that the branded product is better than the same product unlabeled (Branthwaite 2002, Shiv et al. 2005).

If commercial features of day-to-day stuff in our world influence our perceptions of those things, it is no surprise that commercial features also influence medicine. Battles between branded pharmaceuticals and generic competitors are not in name only. Style and color matters in all things of fashion so why not in drugs? Red, yellow and orange are apparently perceived as stimulants, blue and green as tranquilizing, although not consistently (de Craen et al. 1996). More expensive medicine is reported to be better medicine (Waber 2008). Similarly, Cabernet Sauvignon wine labeled as more expensive is reported to be more pleasant than the same wine at a lower price, and differences in the brain can be correlated with differences in pleasantness, just as neural correlates are attributed to placebo (Plassmann et al. 2008). Advertising has been linked by analogy to hypnosis and suggestion, as placebo has. For instance Gould (1991) constructs the notion of advertising suggestion.

Now consider music. To the extent that music acts like a drug, could it possibly be another phenomenon within the broad ambit of placebo? One example is the claim that digital music can produce the effects of illicit recreational drugs. A professor of neuroscience at McGill University in Montreal is reported to have said, "What I think they're actually feeling is a psychological suggestion or a placebo effect" (Banerjee 2010).

The combination of sounds, advertising and suggestion are found together in the advertised benefits of self-help recordings. Repeated subliminal messages from audio recordings have been touted as remedies for a wide variety of problems, hence their use in smoking cessation, memory improvement and weight loss programs. According to neuroscientist Sergio Della Sala (1999), "Having made the commitment and the financial investment, the simple belief that the purchased tapes might work can be sufficient to change beliefs or even to change habits." He calls this the so-called placebo effect.

Placebo is also used by analogy in the context of technology and design. A placebo button is technology that only gives the illusion of control, such as a close-door button in an elevator or a crosswalk button at a pedestrian crossing. For instance Luo (2004) writes that most pedestrian buttons in New York are disconnected and have only imaginary benefit. The comparison to a sugar pill is easy to make: a disconnected crosswalk button does nothing but please the waiting pedestrian.

The effect of laws on behavior has been called a legal placebo effect (Aviram 2006). The claim is that laws manipulate perceptions and thereby overstate or understate the actual benefits of laws. For instance, laws related to airport security may change behavior based on perceptions of airport security as well as actual airport security. A similar notion of meaningless information that changes behavior has emerged in psychology. Weisberg et al. (2008) say that irrelevant "placebic" explanations expressed in terms of neuroscience appear to make people feel better about the explanations. Perhaps placebic explanations of placebo in terms of neuroscience make people feel better about placebo.

These examples from the realms of sport, entertainment, advertising, technology, law and psychology further suggest that there is no sensible boundary around the metaphorical placebo. Or perhaps you can conclude from these examples that there should be no limit to the reach of the marvelous placebo beyond medicine, that placebo is all around us and is an even more useful notion the broader its expanse. Then you have the problem of distinguishing these universal placebos from everyday beliefs, hopes, expectations, superstitions and so on. What distinguishes fake pills and injections from coaching, cheerleading, musical sounds, brand labels, laws, regulations and pushbuttons? It is not always clear whether the placebo metaphor is used by analogy in non-medical examples, or whether medical placebo is actually taken to be the same kind of thing as non-medical placebo, or whether every human activity is ultimately considered to be medical. If putting all of these and many other things in the placebo box seems absurd, however, then maybe the problem is that none of them, including placebo itself, are meaningfully captured by the notion of placebo.

Language upgrades cannot reboot placebo

To use a computing metaphor, many authorities call for upgrades to placebo language. It's as if placebo 2.0 and then maybe 2.1, if not 2.1.1 could work better and offer more user-friendly features than the old placebo 1.0. Suggested upgrades to placebo effect language include self-healing, non-specific effects, context effects (Di Blasi et al. 2001), interpersonal healing (Miller et al. 2009), contextual healing (Miller and Kaptchuk 2008a), meaning response (Brody 1980, Moerman 2003), meaning context and learning response (Jonas 2011), remembered wellness (Benson and Friedman 1996), care effect (Louhiala and Puustinen 2008) and various others. Another approach is to add precision, for instance by subdividing the notion into true and perceived placebo effects (Ernst and Resch 1995) or separating out a placebo effect maximising group (Hróbjartsson 1996).

These are valiant attempts to preserve a placebo category in our language and theory. But there is danger in painting over the flawed placebo with a fresh new logo and brand name or expanding it to include new observations without a revolutionary change to the underlying product. Placebo 1.0 and all of its successors are ill-conceived bug-ridden programs. While it may be satisfying to create a new name, we need more. Labeling something placebo-ish, placebo-like, or placebo-related may foreclose further inquiry into new views.

9 Placebo For Your Thoughts

Placebo effects are often construed as effects of mind on body. But the term placebo is also used when treating conditions of the mind, as if placebo effects are also self-referent effects of mind on mind. For instance, having devoted a chapter of their history of the placebo to a review of psychotherapy, Shapiro and Shapiro (1997) conclude only that it remains to be seen whether psychotherapy is more than placebo. The most sweeping claims, which have been vigorously debated, are that all forms of psychotherapy are equally effective and that all psychotherapies are no more than interchangeable placebos (Luborsky et al. 1975, Jopling 2008).

For conditions treated by the psy-disciplines, the assumption appears to be that anything will do as long as the patient and provider are willing to be deceived by the placebo treatment. Any treatment for the common cold cannot be interchangeable with any treatment for depression or cancer, however, so what is the sense of saying that chicken soup for the common cold is in the same category named placebo as a visit to a psychotherapist or a water injection for cancer? Treatment recipients may have learned different things from their previous experiences with doctors, clinics and health care, and so have different responses and tolerances for fakery, and show different results from the treatments. The possible confounders are endless in kind and number. To talk of psy-placebo and placebo effects, without further distinction, rather than the methods, substances, conditions and interactions in the particular context, leaves them as mysterious as ever.

Reductio ad suggestium

As noted at the outset, placebo is often described as a mental process taking the form of the power of suggestion that helps the suffering person to expect improvement. For instance, Kirsch (1999b) writes:

> The data presented in this paper indicate that hypnotic responses and placebo effects share a common mechanism, that of response expectancy. They share a common mechanism because they are subsets of a broader phenomenon: the phenomenon of suggestion.

Postulating a close link between suggestion and placebo is a departure from earlier research that considered suggestion, placebo and hypnosis to be more independent. For Kirsch, placebo effects are the consequence of expectancy and expectancy is a kind of suggestion. One difference between placebo suggestion and hypnotic suggestion, however, is that the fakery of placebo is intended to fool the subject, whereas hypnotic suggestion takes place in full view of the subject. With placebo, what's going on covertly appears to be authentic, while with hypnosis what's going openly appears to be imaginary.

A generation earlier, another expert on hypnosis wrote, "Suggestion can be defined as the uncritical acceptance of an idea. It is the process by which sensory impressions are conveyed in a meaningful manner to evoke altered psychophysiologic responses. One cannot necessarily equate suggestion with hypnosis unless the latter is accompanied by diversion" (Kroger 1977). Kroger further specified:

> Although suggestion and hypnosis are related to the placebo effect and have much in common, they differ from each other in some ways. The difference is analogous to the comparison made between religious and hypnotic healing. Healing by hypnosis requires belief in the validity of the induction of hypnosis, that is, in the "power" of the hypnotist. Cortical inhibition produced by misdirection of attention is common in hypnosis but not in placebo administration. Faith in the placebo merely indicates faith achieved by previously invoked belief in all drugs as well as the prestige of the physician. Here there is a proper mind-set, based on a high degree of enthusiasm or motivation, belief, confidence, and an expectant attitude.

Going back farther in time, Harrington (2008) says the power of suggestion is a century-old narrative in our culture, with many of its elements being much older. She traces the origins of the power of suggestion through a succession of notions including possession, exorcism, animal magnetism, magnetic somnambulism and hypnotism. In her story-telling view of suggestion, Harrington says the narrative:

> ... invariably begins by introducing at least two characters: a vulnerable, naïve, or needy person (often a patient, quite often a woman) and an authority figure (typically a doctor, healer, hypnotist, or priest, and invariably a man) who is believed to possess either personal charisma, special skills, powerful

medicines, or expert knowledge that brooks no skepticism. If he says something will happen it will!

It is not possible here to delve as deeply into the notion of suggestion as into the notion of placebo. For present purposes, it is enough to question whether suggestion and suggestibility are any more tractable than the concept of placebo that they purportedly explain. As Tasso and Pérez (2008) state:

> Suggestibility is not one thing. Someone cannot be said to be suggestible or nonsuggestible, nor does it seem appropriate to refer to waking or nonwaking suggestibility. This nomenclature is nondescriptive at best, and probably meaningless.

The mysterious notion of suggestion in any event does not provide a firmer foundation for the notion of placebo. Placebo inevitably seems to rest on something else, such as context, expectancy, meaning or suggestion which rests on something else, such as suggestibility and acceptance of an idea, that circles back to rest on placebo. Mikkel Borch-Jacobsen (2009) goes so far as to say that hypnosis stands on suggestion that stands on the unconscious and that none of these constructs, hypnosis, suggestion or the unconscious, have any solid conceptual foundation. To say that placebo is suggestion builds a shaky tower of fragile black boxes one upon another.

Reductio ad placitum

Imagine a world in which physicians are equally effective whether they are trusted, warm and caring or untrusted, cold and uncaring. Assume there is no difference to the patient whether a medical professional takes a detailed history and expresses a personal interest in the patient's life or merely skims over the chart and leaves the room after a minute or two without connecting with the patient eye to eye. Assume also that each suffering person responds equally to physicians and non-physicians, whether they are dressed in crisp white coats or bloody butcher's aprons, whether they are in the awe-inspiring setting of a huge metropolitan teaching hospital or in a tiny rural outpost. In this imaginary world the only things that matter in medicine are the powerful chemicals in drugs together with the physics of sharp instruments and other matters of a mechanical nature.

Authority does not matter in this scenario, so when you are told by an expert that a treatment will help, you have no special reason to believe that it will. In this imaginary world, words of comfort don't matter either. You feel no better if people smile and say you're looking better today than if they frown and say you look worse than ever. Your disease is a separate entity from you and it isn't listening. Assume that neither you nor your disease can be moved by mere words, so your mental and emotional states have no bearing on your medical condition.

Assume that your body reacts to disease in the same way regardless of your learning and experience, conditioned or otherwise. Assume your fears and discomforts have no role to play, so you have no different reaction when the needle pricks your skin whether you are awake or unconscious, or whether you remember the last time it happened and anticipate the pain. The acts of swallowing a pill, receiving an injection or having surgery would not in themselves influence the outcome. In this strange scenario, people are no more sensitive to their treatment than are machines.

People, however, including the bodies they inhabit, are sensitive to words of authority and other aspects of their environment. There is no reason to invoke a mysterious notion of placebo to distinguish people from machines.

Would thinking machines show placebo effects?

Musing about machines as a way of understanding humans has a long history. Descartes, for example, classically considered human automatons as he worked out his distinction between humans with souls and the animals he viewed as machines. To invert the biomedical machine metaphor, that likens bodies and minds to machines, consider the possibility of placebo effects in actual computers and robotic devices.

Does this sound like a ridiculous idea, that the notion of placebo would have anything to do with an electronic device? This idea could at best be premature to consider in a practical sense, given the state of technology now and for some time to come. To the extent that placebo is a medical concept, machines appear to be outside the scope of medicine and placebo. Although computers and robotic devices can perform remarkably in specific domains, such as playing chess or piano, they have yet to achieve the generalized powers of humans. Supposing they could think, nevertheless they don't have bodies in the sense that living organisms do. Without bodies they can't provide a direct analogy to mind-body or brain-body phenomena. Still, this thought experiment highlights various problems with the placebo concept.

Consider an overly simple view for a moment, without getting sidetracked by thorny questions about the nature of consciousness and thought. Machines break and need repairs but they do not yet regenerate their own tissues as living organisms do. Placebo effects are attributes of patients, not the products of repair shops. But assume that some machines could direct their own operations. If a machine could monitor its own functioning, detect malfunctions and repair itself, that would begin to narrow the distinction between broken machine and sick human.

Say for the moment that, in addition to being able to repair themselves, some machines could request repair by other more specialized machines. Perhaps dedicated doctor machines could attend to worker machines. Then a self-repairing machine, perhaps with the help of a doctor machine, would need some criteria by which it determined that it needed repair. It would also have to determine when it had been restored to a state no longer needing repair. If conscious beliefs and expectations are primary drivers behind placebo, then a thinking machine with beliefs and expectations might direct its own repair based on its beliefs and expectations. Those beliefs and expectations might influence the criteria for needing repair and for restoration to proper functioning. Unconscious conditioning is also part of placebo theory. We could assume that a thinking machine had conscious and unconscious events, but that is not necessary for placebo effects based on belief and expectation.

We have only begun to explore the intersection of placebo and machines. This thought experiment could be extended to many other aspects of thinking machines. For instance, we could delve into the criteria used by a thinking machine to determine whether it needs repair. In that regard, since placebo and pain are often associated, we could draw machine analogies with pain. Then we could follow the well-trodden path of speculation about whether machines could ever feel pain, which Dennett (1978) conspicuously denied, sparking a vigorous debate.

But why? What do we gain? The placebo metaphor is a stretch for machines as it is for humans. All of these references to placebo in relation to thinking machines are unnecessary. The future of self-repairing machines and doctor devices that fix other devices can be better described without the notion of placebos and placebo effects. Placebo only adds an extra layer of complication that is not inherent in the relations of machines or humans to their own states of repair.

Unexplained cure, unexplained harm

While placebos may be the most common cures in medicine, medically unexplained symptoms may be the most common complaints: "Medically unexplained symptoms of pain and bodily dysfunction are the single most prevalent class of symptoms in primary care" (Henningsen et al. 2003). Putting these two observations together, does that mean the mystery of the most common cure is related to the mystery of the most prevalent unexplained symptoms?

Rarely included in discussions of placebo or nocebo is a cluster of phenomena gathered under the category of somatoform disorders or somatization. Related terms include somatization disorder, pain disorder, conversion disorder, hypochondriasis and body dysmorphic disorder (Lamberty 2008). For the purposes of this discussion, the common element is that somatizing patients have a history of unexplained symptoms that seem to have no discernable physical basis.

Unexplained symptoms raise questions related to placebo and nocebo. For instance, is somatization itself a subcategory of nocebo? To the extent that there is debate about whether placebos can cure disease or illness or both, are somatoform disorders also parseable into the same divisions? As with the mysteries of placebo, somatization also highlights how little is known about the relationship between mind (or brain) and body.

For the purposes of this discussion, if both unexplained symptoms and unexplained cures are involved in a large proportion of medical cases, both of which are closely linked with placebo and nocebo, even if they are not the same symptoms or cures, we can stop saying placebo or nocebo and start saying of the unexplained: I don't kow.

10 Placebo Blind

As noted early in this discussion, it is curious that the placebo-controlled clinical trial has become a standard for medical science when placebo itself remains so mysterious and is anything but standard. Placebo is not subject to the same standards as the drugs that are tested in placebo-controlled trials (Golomb 1995, Golomb et al. 2010). Practically anything goes in the strange do-it-yourself domain of decoy drugs, such as hiding tablets inside capsules to compensate for an improperly prepared supply that didn't match the drug (van Reekum 2010).

To label something as a placebo control is not sufficiently informative about what is compared in any particular experiment. Nor does the label placebo control provide assurance that the experiment was placebo-controlled, whatever that may mean. Consider the example of olive oil used as a placebo in a drug trial for heart disease. It was reported in these terms (Scottish Society 1971):

> A trial is reported of the effects of giving clofibrate to prevent progression of pre-existing ischaemic heart disease. There were two groups randomly distributed between clofibrate (350 patients) and placebo (367 patients) regimens.

The authors claim that they compared a drug with a placebo. Does that mean this is a placebo-controlled trial of the difference between an inert treatment and an active biomedical treatment? The detailed part of the report of the trial design reveals that the placebo was "olive oil dispensed in identical capsules." Nobody could replicate that placebo control in another experiment since we don't know any details of the capsules or their contents, such as whether it was virgin, cold-pressed or any other specific formulation of olive oil from a specific vendor or region, because the report provides no more description than "olive oil." Much evidence suggests that olive oil is not an inert substance in the cardiovascular system. For instance, Covas (2007) reviews research on olive oil and the cardiovascular system and finds a wide range of beneficial effects. We don't know if the results would have been different if the control treatment had been corn oil or some other vegetable oil or some other substance altogether that resembled clofibrate capsules enough to fool people.

A more recent example of questionable placebo controls is provided by a small pilot study of psilocybin treatment for anxiety in cancer patients (Grob et al. 2010). The placebo in that experiment was niacin in 250mg capsules. The authors say, "A niacin placebo was chosen because it often induces a mild physiological reaction (eg, flushing) without altering the psychological state." Flushing and other well-known cutaneous effects of niacin could produce anxiety in unsuspecting subjects, but more problematic is evidence that niacin can relieve anxiety symptoms. Niacin may not be inert and therefore may not be an appropriate control in the context of treating anxiety, but absent standards for placebo experiments, nobody can say.

Similarly the placebo used in a trial of irritable bowel syndrome was avicel, microcrystalline cellulose, what the authors themselves describe as "a common inert excipient for pharmaceuticals" (Kaptchuk et al. 2010). The cellulose was delivered in blue and maroon gelatin capsules. Avicel is common, but by the standards of evidence-based medicine, we would need randomized controlled trials to determine whether cellulose filler is inert in a medical condition partly constituted by symptoms such as fullness that might be influenced by cellulose with potential laxative properties, and whether blue and maroon capsules had any significance different from, say, red, yellow or white.

We need to know why the experimenters believe that these are valid dummy controls, that olive oil has no effect on heart disease, or that niacin has no effect on anxiety, or that cellulose filler passes through the body inertly without influencing the very syndrome under investigation. Researchers should provide a rigorous justification for the the specific choice of control, such as the type and quantity of olive oil and not some other olive oil or some other control altogether, and not protect it under the general cloak called placebo. If they were to provide additional evidence of the effects of that type of control treatment on the outcome, then not only would the controls improve but researchers might also be prompted to investigate sooner whether olive oil treatment influences heart disease, whether vitamins affect anxiety or other potential consequences of the selected control treatment.

Knowledge-controlled, expectation-induced

To unwind the placebo knots tied up with clinical trials, we must look in detail at the methodology of blinding. Blinding, as in a double-blind clinical trial in which participants don't know who got what treatment, is another instance in which placebo language gets in the way. In this usage the word blinding is a metaphor for not knowing. Terminology associated with blinding shares some of the problems of placebo, both blinding and placebo being variously and ambiguously used even among experts (Devereaux 2001, Schulz et al. 2002).

In the present discussion, it is important to note that blinding of participants in randomized controlled trials is not just a method for counteracting placebo effects but rather is a more general method of influencing knowledge and belief. Also note that the word participants in some discussions of blinding is arbitrarily limited to experimental subjects. In this discussion, participants include everyone participating, not just people who swallow pills, but also investigators, caregivers, statisticians, writers and anyone else whose participation influences what happens throughout an experiment.

Blinding (sometimes called masking) has a long and complex history. Kaptchuk (1998) divides the history of blinding into five phases from early attempts to detect fraud through to current methodology that combines the intentional ignorance techniques of blinding with randomization in the randomized double-blind clinical trial. Introduction of the now hallowed term double-blind has been attributed to Harry Gold who advocated the advantages of double-blind methodology. Although use of blindfolds in experiments has been traced back through the centuries, one of Gold's colleagues suggested that they may have used the term blind test merely because of an advertising campaign for Old Gold cigarettes in which blindfolded smokers compared cigarette brands (Shapiro and Shapiro 1997). Currently the legacy of Harry Gold and perhaps Old Gold has been elevated to the gold standard in evidence-based medicine that, for its critics, has become a golden calf (Kaptchuk 2001).

Given the impracticality of physically blindfolding everyone to keep them ignorant of interventions, experimenters often use clever tricks, such as specially constructed pills, as magicians control knowledge about the rabbit hidden in the specially constructed hat, without physically blinding the audience. Trickery is not of the essence, however, in the sense of being a necessary and sufficient experimental condition. Fake treatment is not sufficient to conceal knowledge when effects of the experimental treatment are detectably different from effects of the fake treatment. Some treatments are too different to be interchangeable and others simply cannot be faked. There is also some evidence that patients can be satisfied even if they are told the treatment is fake (Park and Covi 1965, Jopling 2008, Egeth 2009, Kaptchuk et al. 2010). Fake treatment also is not necessary when the same experimental treatment is delivered to everyone while knowledge is controlled by delivering different information, as in open-hidden methods during which all patients receive the same drug but are told different stories about the treatment.

In the example of treatments delivered in pill form, people can hardly be fooled if they're not given any pills at all, so they have to be given something that makes them think they're being treated. Depending on the circumstances, including aims of the experiment, costs and availability of alternatives, they might be given pills constructed from powerful drugs that have both wanted and unwanted effects, or constructed from less powerful drugs with less obvious effects, or from substances intended to mimic only the harmful effects of powerful drugs, or from substances intended to do nothing but fool them. They could be given multiple treatments at the same time, for instance one pill without the experimental drug and another pill with the drug.

These different constructions and combinations, illustrating only some of numerous possible interventions, are obscured by lumping some constructions in the category called placebo, or in a variant category such as active placebo. The curiously named active placebo is not an inactive do-nothing placebo but a fake drug pretending to be a drug, that is, a doubly fake "fake placebo" (Park and Covi 1965). Placebo terminology of any kind, however, is not needed to describe what are now called double-blind placebo-controlled trials.

The notion of placebo imports an unnecessarily mysterious and uncontrollable quality to the distinctly not mysterious deliberate construction of experimental interventions. They are specially controlled interventions in experiments designed to produce specific observed outcomes and exclude other outcomes when compared in various combinations. Things compared in randomized controlled trials cannot be equated with Beecher's powerful placebos that mysteriously reduce suffering in clinical patients. Trials are deliberately arranged to be unlike clinical practice in which knowledge is uncontrolled, and both providers and recipients of medical care usually know who gets what treatment and continually adjust their mutual beliefs and expectations in context.

Trial participants can often guess who is receiving fake treatment. Despite the best efforts of research methodologists, their subjects and experimenters are not easily tricked. The more potent the intervention, the more apparent are the detected differences compared to less potent interventions. Investigators may detect traces of the experimental drug in clinical examinations and laboratory test results. Patients may suffer from side effects. To reduce differences detected from these and other clues, researchers could try to make the compared interventions more alike. For instance, they could mimic the harmful effects of an experimental drug with some other substance, the fake placebo, that does not contain the drug but tries to behave like the drug. But creating an active placebo that has identical effects to a potent drug is almost impossible. "To obtain a truly double blind experiment, each patient would have to receive a placebo with the same physiological effects as the medication produces in each patient" (Ney 1986). The more potent the intervention, the less likely it is to be blind and the more difficult it is to claim that the trial was actually blind.

The experimental drug could also be constructed with less powerful effects to minimize detectable differences from other interventions in the experiment. Drugs that do little or nothing are more easily masked than potent drugs, but the point of a trial is to detect differences not to make the interventions appear to be the same. Detecting differences is desirable. Pharmaceutical manufacturers want their products to be detectably different from less effective treatments. Failure to blind does not necessarily mean failure of the experiment but could mean the opposite, that the trial showed detectable differences. If trial participants can accurately guess who got what treatment, that may be good evidence that the treatments actually are different, and ultimately that the experimental drug works.

It is important to emphasize that blinding is an issue of controlling knowledge, while belief and expectation are not so easily controlled. Randomized double-blind trials use various methods to prevent everyone from knowing what intervention is actually allocated. Still, everyone has beliefs and expectations about what might be the case, notwithstanding their knowledge. They believe and expect various things about their moment-to-moment existence, their future and their memories, some of which may be based on knowledge, some of which may be based on feelings, intuitions, misapprehensions, fallacious reasoning and many other grounds. To the extent that beliefs and expectations influence outcomes, blinding does not erase or equalize these factors in clinical trials. Indeed, blinding itself might be the source of a recursive bias resulting from the participant's awareness of being in a blind trial (Kaptchuk 2001). Blinding, like randomization, has become such a dogmatic standard, formalized in the randomized double-blind trial, that it is easy to forget that neither methodology has magical powers to generate meaningful unbiased experimental observations (Benedetti 2007, Worrall 2007).

Consider the debates about assessment of blinding in clinical trials (Fergusson et al. 2004, Sackett 2007). One view is represented by those who want evidence that participants actually were blind throughout the trial. They say trial participants should be asked what they knew or could guess about who got what treatment.

Another view is preferred by those who may acknowledge the laudatory goal of proving that everyone was ignorant of treatment allocation, but who nevertheless raise questions about whether and how the goal might be achieved. They say we can't tell if guesses influenced outcomes or outcomes influenced guesses. For instance, can we assess blinding in experiments by simply asking participants after the trial to guess what treatment was received? An experimental subject's reasoning might be, "It worked. So I must have been given the new drug." The researcher's reasoning might be, "This group had better outcomes than the other group, and since my hypothesis is that the new drug is the better treatment, this must be the group that got the new drug." Those answers reveal less about blinding than about fallacies and human reasoning. This situation is analogous to asking the magician's audience to offer guesses about the rabbit and the hat, which guesses depend as much on their background knowledge and theories about magic as on the particular performance, rabbit or hat.

Everyone participating in the experiment may be prevented from knowing who got what intervention, but being smart talking primates who can see patterns in the mere arrangements of stars, people still have ideas about what's happening to them and around them. Beliefs and the biases they support are not just to be buried in randomized controlled trials but are to be investigated in their own right. After best efforts to control knowledge, accounting for these other influences remains problematic. "I didn't know" who got what treatment may be the ideal answer from the perspective of blinding but the actual case may be "I didn't know but I hoped" or "I suspected but I pretended" or "I wasn't fooled" or even "I knew but I lied."

Testing for blinding is only a part of the overall question whether the experiment was properly conducted, and such methodological considerations are only part of what influences the experimental result. Failure of blinding is only one influence on belief and not the most significant one. A more general approach in medicine after placebo is to inquire generally into the sources of beliefs, expectations, hopes and related contextual influences. Ignorance of who got what intervention partly addresses issues of knowledge.

But if hope, belief and expectation influence the outcome, in some ways for experimental subjects, in other ways for experimenters, and in still other ways for interactions among them, then the question is not whether blinding was maintained but what were participants' beliefs, expectations and hopes.

Given the complex interactions of knowledge, belief, expectation, hope and so on, it is no wonder that blinding is often oversimplified even by experts. There seems to be an implicit preference for simple binary assessments (whether the experiment was double-blind or not), over multiple possibilities (such as double-blind, not double-blind, maybe, don't know), that may in turn be more tractable but less informative than complex answers such as:

> Before the trial I didn't think much about placebos but when they asked me to guess if I was getting placebos and to tell them how confident I was in my answer I figured it was important, and at the beginning I was worried that I was only getting the placebo but then I thought it was the drug, but then I wasn't sure and after a while I figured it really didn't matter because nothing else worked before anyway but I still hoped it would.

Discrete, quantitative categories are easier to deal with than subjective, qualitative, non-linear narrative that rambles over the person's past, present and future. Controlled trials are attempts to eliminate subjective factors, in preference for the elusive objectivity of science, but subjectivity, to use a hydraulic metaphor, is not infinitely compressible and will eventually leak out somewhere.

Blinding, and the use of trickery to control knowledge, is sometimes wrapped up with the problem of deception. Consider an experiment reported by Kirsch and Weixel (1988) who distinguish blinding from deception. They use the notion of blinding when referring to the standard clinical trial in which subjects are informed that the treatment may be a placebo or a drug.

They consider deception to be the case in which the subject receives placebo but is led to believe it is a drug. By contrast, Miller and Kaptchuk (2008b) interpret deception more broadly to include using only a placebo for all subjects when they are told they may receive placebo or medication (so that for patients expecting either placebo or drug, deliberately giving placebo is deceptive but randomly doing so is acceptable).

Deception, as interpreted by Kirsch and Weixel, more closely compares with the clinical situation in which patients believe the treatment is effective, rather than the experimental trial situation, in which subjects believe they may or may not be receiving an effective treatment. In their experiment they gave decaffeinated coffee to every subject, with some led to believe it could be caffeinated or decaffeinated and others led to believe that it was a well-known brand of caffeinated coffee. They measured subjective mood (feelings of alertness, relaxation, tension), predictions of performance and retrodictions about whether the coffee actually had caffeine, as well as physical parameters including reaction time, pulse rate and blood pressure. Although as hypothesized the deceived group showed some greater effects, the two groups had some opposite results that may have been influenced by the subjects' relative uncertainty about what they were drinking. Consequently Kirsch and Weixel recommend that an ideal experiment should test all four combinations of treatment and information about the treatment, that is: give the drug and say they're getting the drug, give no drug but say they're getting the drug, give the drug but say it's not the drug, give no drug and say they're not receiving the drug.

A different approach to the problems of blinding and deception was used in what the authors say is the first reported clinical trial to compare "open-label placebo" with no treatment (Kaptchuk et al. 2010). Eighty patients with irritable bowel syndrome received either no treatment or placebo pills openly described as placebos. So there were no groups comparable to the above "give this but say it's that" groups. In particular, there were no groups who just took the pills without being influenced by the suggestion that placebos are powerful. The experimenters encouraged all patients to believe in the power of placebos and those who took them reported marginally better subjective outcomes than the untreated. The authors acknowledge various limitations of this unblind study but nevertheless conclude that placebos administered without deception may be effective treatment for irritable bowel syndrome.

The emphasis here is not on resolving ethical debates about the propriety of deception in experiments, or to set methodological standards, but only to point out that those debates are not necessarily or even helpfully conceived in terms of placebo. In medicine after placebo, experimenters preferably can report in detail exactly what was compared and in what combinations together with what information. To say something was compared with placebo implies some but not other of the multiple meanings of placebo, with possible confusions among meanings relating to experiments and meanings that allude to mysterious mind-body medicine. But controlled trials use knowledge control to eliminate, not to investigate, mysterious influences. A placebo control, such as a sugar pill, is supposed to neutralize the mind-body problem in an experiment. But there is no linear equation with separate terms for mind (or brain) and body that can be altered independently. The mind feeds back to the body that feeds back to the mind.

To summarize the intersection of blinding in experiments with medicine after we stop saying placebo: experiments can be partly controlled by knowledge control and information framing, but the uncontrolled beliefs, hopes, expectations, guesses, hunches, suspicions, doubts and prejudices of all participants are influenced by many sources in addition to knowledge, and at no time is the notion of placebo needed to say so. All of these complexities may be relevant matters but they can be reasonably well described without saying placebo, active placebo, placebo effects or placebo-related effects.

But what do you say to those who want a handle attached to what we now call placebo controls and who argue that placebo is as good a word as any? The following suggestions represent only one tentative prescription among the many creative solutions that others will surely find. Instead of saying it's a double-blind experiment with placebo control, say that you are trying to set the same beliefs and expectations in everyone while giving them different treatments. Instead of saying this is the placebo control group, say exactly what treatment they are getting, how they are being informed and treated and what they report of their hopes, beliefs and expectations. Account for the differences between belief in the effects of a treatment, in the possibility of getting a treatment and knowledge of being in an experiment. Detail what participants in a control group are getting instead of the experimental treatment and provide grounds for the claim that they can be fooled. Provide evidence that the trick actually worked in this particular group. Such evidence may be conceived more broadly than just questioning participants before, during or after experiments to assess blinding. Ask and report generally about matters of communication, beliefs, expectations and hopes, and their influence on outcomes.

With the focus removed from the mysterious placebo, and with recognition that beliefs and expectations are difficult to control, eventually these experiments may come to be known as knowledge-controlled trials, expectation-induced trials or even belief-altered narratives, or by other terms that may evolve along with current theory, instead of double-blind placebo-controlled or open-hidden placebo-related trials.

11 Post-Placebo

When Western medicine abandoned the idea that there are four fundamental things called humors, physicians continued to observe bodily fluids. But those fluids were re-conceived in terms other than humors and their roles in relation to other medical conceptions were revised. The old terms were abandoned, so we no longer see the same yellow bile, black bile, phlegm and blood that according to the numerology of the times were viewed in relation to many other conceptual quartets, including the four seasons, the four elements (fire, earth, water and air), the four organs (liver, spleen, brain and heart), the four qualities (hot, dry, cold and moist) and the four temperaments (choleric, melancholic, phlegmatic and sanguine). Similarly after we abandon placebo we can continue to see various kinds of medical interventions correlated with changes in the brain and body without seeing placebos and placebo effects.

Or consider an example that shows the opposite of no longer seeing an old thing but rather seeing something that was not there before. Only a generation ago the accepted explanation for gastric ulcers was expressed in terms of stress and diet. Bacteria were invisible in the explanatory story. Now that condition has been revised in terms of germ theory, so when we think of gastric ulcers, the story includes bacteria in addition to personality, behavior and lifestyle. Similarly in medicine after placebo, new possibilities will appear.

When we stop using placebo terminology we will not leave behind all uses in medical research and clinical practice of the sugar pills and water injections of placebo lore. In medicine after placebo, there will still be sugar pills and water, but we won't see placebos. We won't see placebo effects, either, just as we no longer see Galen's mysterious faculties for pulsation in the arteries, that made sense when the heart was believed to be a heater and therefore unrelated to pulsating arteries. Now no mysterious arterial effects need explanation since the heart is conceived as a pump. Similarly, the mysterious conception of placebo effects and their connections to other medical conceptions will be re-examined.

What do you say if not placebo?

What you say when you don't say placebo is similar to what you don't say of other old medical notions. A new generation grows up wondering how anyone could have believed in the old notions and the next generation forgets them.

You probably don't now think in terms of melancholic or phlegmatic patients, for instance. Nor are you likely to search for replacements for the old medical term vital spirits. If we look for a one-to-one correspondence between old and new, between placebo and its replacement, we are only rearranging the conceptual furniture. Instead the whole placebo construct needs to be torn down and a new structure built up, so that in future we won't even see the old structure, as today's medicine does not see the structures of ancient medicine.

Placebo-free language

We are so used to the placebo concept that its absence would seem to leave a gap in our language. But removing placebo would no more leave a gap than removing debris from an ocean would leave a gap in the water. Placebo is a relatively new word for observations that have been and can be expressed without using the language of placebo. For instance, consider this statement from more than a century ago by the German physician Albert Moll:

People who suffer from sleeplessness have often been sent to sleep by taking something which they were told was a sleeping draught, but which was really some inert substance. They slept because they expected to do so. When they learn that the medicine is not a sleeping draught they no longer expect sleep, and do not sleep (Moll 1891).

Moll does not mention placebo. The label placebo was not needed then and is not needed now. We understand the observations that Moll was describing without the intermediary layer of placebo. Moreover, he relies on the concept of expectation as we do today. Placebo-free language apparently has changed little in the past century. It's placebo language that causes problems.

Mr Wright sans placebo

Return now to the dramatic story of Mr Wright's temporary reprieve from cancer that has been repeated in the literature as a remarkable example of the placebo effect. Can his story be told without placebo? The anecdote as reported by Klopfer (1957) actually does not use the word placebo. It refers to such treatments and influences as oxygen, injections, faith and fanfare, but not placebo. There is no need to add a layer with the placebo on top of unexplained correlation.

Absent a placebo viewpoint, Mr Wright's anecdote shrinks like his tumors, from a unique, improbable, inflated example of the power of placebo to a common anecdote about one of the few certain medical events, namely death. Mr Wright's condition fluctuated during treatment. Then he died. From the available evidence, we don't know much more than that. There's no need to invoke the mysterious placebo explanation to say: I don't know.

Clinical trials could be symmetrical

Things compared with experimental treatments in clinical trials include standard treatments, placebos, and no treatment, among other variations. The main question in a trial is usually whether the experimental treatment is superior to, equivalent to, or at least not worse than the things compared with it. The focus of clinical trials is not the control group which is generally regarded as if it need not be investigated and reported in detail.

This seems too obvious to point out. Why would the control group be the focus of an experiment anyway? The whole idea is to test the experimental treatment, not to test the control treatment. After all, the sponsor of the trial usually wants to show that the experimental treatment works and therefore should be made generally available for patients.

In medicine after placebo, accounts of things compared in trials could become symmetrical, with as much concern for theories and explanations of control treatments as for the experimental treatment, and for people and their beliefs as for their bodies. Experimenters, and medical professionals in general, could value rather than attempt to exclude beliefs and expectations. Theories and explanations of control treatments could be as detailed and debated as theories and explanations of experimental treatments. Observations of people would include measures of their feelings, beliefs and expectations, not just impersonal parameters such as heart rate and blood pressure.

In a symmetrical post-placebo view, the things compared could be equally scrutinized. Experimenters would have as good an explanation backing the action or non-action of the controls as of the experimental treatment. Not a black box explanation, such as merely reporting that they used a placebo or active control, but a formal explanation as rigorous as the explanation given for the experimental treatment. To claim that the control treatment appeared identical to the experimental treatment is not enough. For instance, experimenters would explain why they chose the particular form, color, size and treatment regimen for their experimental and control treatments and how they determined that these and related choices had minimal uncontrolled influences on the outcomes.

Symmetry would apply to beliefs and expectations of everyone involved in the clinical trial. Currently the emphasis in clinical trials is on the things compared, not on the people involved. Questions about the person have been limited to issues such as whether the trial was properly blind or masked to avoid biases. Absent the notion of placebo, there could be more symmetrical interest in people and things.

An example of a trial that puts expectation in the forefront is that of Linde et al. (2007) who observed more pain relief among patients with higher expectations, whether they received acupuncture or sham acupuncture. In a post-placebo world questions might include: what did the acupuncturist believe and expect when delivering sham acupuncture? What were the patients' beliefs and expectations regarding the acupuncturist, the procedures and the surroundings? What exactly was said to the participants during the experiment and by whom? Were patients influenced by other patients in addition to the medical staff? Were they influenced by their own online research, as many patients are? These are only some of the questions to explore. What people can't say also matters as much as what they say. Unsaid influences merit their own examination. Expectation and belief are only part of a story that overlaps with culture, learning, conditioning, tacit knowledge, meaning, wants, needs and related terms that would no longer be excluded by concealing them in the placebo box. There is nothing to be gained by labeling any group as the placebo group whether they receive open treatment, hidden treatment, fake treatment or are put on a waiting list or have no involvement in the formal medical system at all.

Language change need not come only from experts. Patients may also have something to offer. For instance, Kaptchuk et al. (2009) provide evidence of the language used by patients in the placebo arm of randomized controlled trials. According to these researchers, who point out that patients' experiences in the placebo arm have not been investigated, patients "almost never endorsed 'expectation' of improvement but spoke of 'hope' instead and frequently reported despair." Yet recent placebo literature is dominated by talk of expectation despite its differences from hope (Miceli and Castelfranchi 2010, Nwoye 2011). Non-experts can contribute solutions to conceptual and terminological problems.

Research funding, training and regulation are some of the other realms that would need to accommodate the passing of placebo and a move toward symmetry. Including patient expectations and related observations implies that clinicians and researchers need to be trained to value and use them. If conditioning and learning mediate changes in health, then we might invoke the weight of our higher institutions of conditioning and learning, including professors, educational authorities, courses and the money that makes them function, to get more from the particular conditioning and learning that makes some people get better. Regulators could change the rules for clinical trials, and in particular look for ways to reduce opportunities for experimenters to influence results by using controls that hide in the black box now called placebo. More funding of post-placebo research will be needed, whether on methodological matters such as investigating expectations, or conducting symmetrical research or training medical professionals and the public.

You have control

Control of oneself and one's environment could be viewed as the essence of human activity. To the extent that placebo is powered by a feeling of control over an uncertain future, almost anything that offers explanation or control can be effective. Actual control is not the only form of control that matters.

In one meaning model of placebo, a central part of meaning is promised control, that is, "holding out an enhanced promise of mastery or control over the symptoms" (Brody 1997). Brody refers to something less controlling than actual control. Promise implies expectation that the desired outcome could be fulfilled, so the notion of control over symptoms is also related to the notion that expectation influences treatment outcomes. Extending that idea further, it's worth exploring whether not only a promise or expectation of actual control but also an illusion of control can be effective.

Illusion of control resembles superstition. Both of these phenomena manufacture order from chance. Whereas superstition is a false pairing of cause and effect, illusion of control is a false belief in being able to cause effects. Through an influential series of studies, Langer (1975) showed that experimental subjects expressed more confidence and expected more success when given an illusion of control over a purely chance outcome. She introduced elements of skill, such as choice and competition, into games of chance by, for instance, letting subjects choose a lottery ticket. Although choice of the ticket had no actual influence on the chance of winning, subjects were more confident that they would win when they had this illusory control. Many other researchers have extended these findings about illusion of control or sense of control. Loss of control can induce a learned helplessness while a sense of control can improve health and quality of life (Rodin 1986).

Instead of saying placebo, we could not only speak in terms of expectations, we could be even more specific about how we use various techniques to alter expectations. We could investigate whether we are increasing sense of control and reducing feelings of helplessness. We could say we are using our understanding of the relationship between control and cure to help patients in clinical practice and to devise experiments in medical research.

Placebo-only therapies

Bausell (2007) concludes a detailed review of complementary alternative medicine (CAM) with these words: "CAM therapies are nothing more than cleverly packaged placebos. And that is almost all there is to say about the science of CAM." In a similar vein, Jopling (2008) considers whether the vast range of psychotherapies are all reliant on placebo effects. The issue here is not whether these authors are correct in concluding that CAM and psychotherapy are powered by placebo. Within the current placebo view, maybe some are and some are not so conceived. The issue is the notion of placebo that is central to their main thesis about the nature of these therapies and the methodology for evaluating them. In medicine after placebo, there is nothing to be gained by describing and evaluating these and other therapies in terms of placebo.

Consider recent debates about whether CAM deserves a special status exempt from the rigors of randomized double-blind placebo-controlled trials. To avoid favoring vested interests and untested orthodoxy, medical researcher Iain Chalmers (1998) advocates a single standard for evaluation of any health care intervention. Psychologist Harald Walach (2001) argues against double-blind placebo-controlled trials of CAM because CAM does not operate only on the magic-bullet model of a specific drug fixing a specific cellular pathology, but in a holistic way. Hansen and Kappel (2010) dismiss arguments that CAM is too holistic or based on principles too different from orthodox medicine to be subjected to the same evidence-based standards. They acknowledge that some people will choose CAM fo religious or philosophical reasons that do not highly value scientific evidence but they argue that state-funded CAM should be tested by randomized controlled trials. Miller et al. (2004) say that CAM should be tested in placebo-controlled trials and that CAM therapies may have value even when shown to be no better than placebo. Complementary medicine expert Edzard Ernst (2009) also says that the principles of evidence-based medicine must be applied to CAM and that there is evidence that some CAM interventions do more good than harm. Medical philosopher Kirstin Borgerson (2005) posits three possible sieves for testing CAM: evidence-based medicine as it is now, or some special status outside of evidence-based medicine or a future improved form of evidence-based medicine with new research designs. She advocates the latter choice. Psychologist Pete Greasley (2010) argues that it is simply absurd to evaluate many CAM therapies, such as reflexology, iridology, and acupuncture, that are based on magical thinking and the fiction of analogical correspondence (as for example the human shape of mandrake root is said to endow it with magical properties).

Those who equate CAM with placebo are telling a causal story about therapy. One version of that story is to say CAM is all placebo in the sense that it does no biomedical causal work and so is interchangeable with any other placebo. Another version is to say that CAM is no better than placebo, which could imply that CAM does some causal work by different means than placebo but only an amount equivalent to placebo. Yet another version is to ignore the details of how the work is done and simply say that CAM is synonymous with placebo however the causal work happens. In any version of the story about comparison between CAM and placebo, we cannot say that the therapy works better than doing nothing or doing something else. For that story, CAM must be compared to doing nothing or doing something else. Then we are faced with the problems of the idealized no-treatment group.

Like dividing medicine between placebo and not placebo, the binary division between medicine and not medicine is another false dichotomy. No clear line delimits where orthodox medicine ends and CAM begins. Perhaps whatever works eventually becomes orthodox medicine. Advocates of CAM and defenders of biomedicine alike can both accuse the other side of false dualism: for instance, to argue that biomedicine ignores the effects of mind on body is at the same time to argue that mind is separate from body. A double standard for assessing whether medical interventions work would be yet another false dichotomy.

Ethics after placebo

Placebo is central to many ethical questions in medicine. Is use of placebos ethical in clinical practice? In clinical trials, is it ethical to use placebos while depriving participants of available treatment? Is the goal of placebo research to find much better treatments, marginally better treatments, equivalent treatments, not worse treatments, more or less profitable treatments, or harmless yet effective treatments? Are the ethics of treatment decisions the same for relatively minor, chronic conditions as for serious, acute, potentially life-threatening conditions? Does placebo use in sport medicine amount to undetectable cheating? After medicine abandons the language of placebo, questions such as these will not disappear but they may be parsed differently.

There will be no need, for instance, to distinguish placebo-controlled trials from active-controlled trials. As this is another false dichotomy associated with placebo, no absolute distinction between them is possible in any event (Howick 2009, Nunn 2009b). There will also be no absolute distinction between informing the patient and assessing the benefit for the patient, since what patients are told influences their beliefs, knowledge and expectations, and may alter the benefits and risks (Miller and Colloca 2011). The features of any control treatment, whether currently called a placebo or not, will be explained to patients and set out in detail when reported by researchers. The focus in medicine after placebo will be on methodologies that do not deprive patients of existing treatment for the sake of increasing knowledge, but rather treat the patient while also providing knowledge. Exploring such problems free from placebo may also provide clearer direction for medical decision-makers.

Additional avenues of research may appear when examining belief directly, rather than as a mechanism of placebo. Belief in relation to the role the person plays may influence a medical outcome. Consider the beliefs of patient and provider. Four possibilities exist, along with an infinite range of degrees of belief and interactions among these four:

—patient and provider believe the intervention works
—patient and provider believe it does not work
—provider believes it works but patient does not
—provider does not believe it works but patient does

More likely the provider and patient have shades of belief, not absolute beliefs in the effectiveness of treatment. They could have a range of commitments to their beliefs, and they could believe that some of the effects could be attributed to their own beliefs. To the extent that these possibilities influence medical outcomes, along with other possibilities including variations on learning and conditioning now described as placebo mechanisms, they can be described and investigated withou the notion of placebo.

In the context of placebo, belief is often discussed as if it were one thing. But belief as the basis for the placebo notion has not been sufficiently explored in relation to different kinds of belief. One notable and widespread species of belief, for example, is religious belief. Although many studies have examined religious belief in the context of medicine, evidence of connections among religion, spirituality, medicine and health is equivocal (Sloan et al. 1999, Pargament and Cummings 2010). Questions that have not been answered include: does a medical provider's religious belief influence patient outcomes? Is a belief in the power of words such as prayer different from belief in the power of words from caregivers and sports coaches? What experimental control group is comparable to a belief group? Is religious belief the same as belief in therapy and if not, how can they be distinguished? The sense of control offered both by promise of cure and by religion could be closely related (Ellison and Burdette 2011). Exploring questions such as these is not helped by looking at them in terms of placebo effects, prayer effects or coaching effects.

An important ethical question concerning placebos is whether placebos should be used at all and if they are, whether they should be used when conventional treatment exists. Both in clinical practice and in medical experiments, views about placebo use range widely. At one extreme are calls for complete prohibition of these ineffective deceptions anywhere in medicine, while at the other extreme placebo advocates want to increase research into and use of these miraculous cures (Hróbjartsson 2008, Louhiala 2009). Some go as far as to argue that placebos are not always deceptive and may even be "morally imperative" (Lichtenberg et al. 2004).

Too often the debate gets caught in the puzzles of placebo terminology. For instance, while arguing against the use of placebos in medical research, Kottow (2010) says, "Research placebos are not placebos at all, for their purpose is not to please the patient but to supposedly satisfy the method of research protocols." Rather than try to convince medical researchers that their placebo controls are not placebos at all, and return us to the quagmire of placebo misunderstanding, let us leave placebo behind to move medical research and practice forward.

Given the current placebo paradigm, how could anyone talk sensibly about placebo ethics without talking in terms of placebo?

Rather than rehearse the voluminous ethical debates about whether to use placebos, consider how the language could change in medicine after placebo. For instance, in clinical practice, we now ask if it is ethical to deceive a patient with a placebo. Absent the notion of placebo, and depending on what models of conditioning ensue, we might ask, for example, whether it is ethical to condition or teach a patient to expect pain relief. Various methodologies could be employed if conditioning or teaching were deemed to be acceptable medicine. In research, where we now ask about the propriety of using a placebo control when a standard treatment exists, we might ask how we can modify expectations and under what circumstances. Models and language of conditioning, learning and expectation are also likely to change as they are freed from their current incarnation as placebo mechanisms. Changing viewpoints opens doors to a changed world.

Patients and placebo-free language

Among the many reasons to advocate for medicine after placebo is that talking in terms of placebo is arguably unethical. Because the placebo concept has so many problems, most patients, if not their providers, cannot practically be informed when medical matters are expressed in terms of placebo. Although experts may claim to understand at least some aspects of placebo, nobody fully understands it, and in any event non-experts involved in medical decisions expressed in terms of placebo must rely on experts and their problematic placebo terminology.

Communication between provider and patient is a complex matter involving many nuances. Given the constrained face-to-face time that patients ordinarily get to spend with their medical professionals, conversation between expert and patient may involve lies of omission and miscommunication as much as lies of commission. By definition, experts know more and have more to say in their field of expertise than non-experts do. Between expert and patient, given limited time and lack of shared knowledge, despite the best of intentions, the expert may never be able to avoid in some respects deceiving the patient.

If experts are puzzled by the notion of placebo, what is the average person or patient to understand, that is not deceptive, about placebo? The answer offered here is that too many problems are inherent in talking to patients about placebo, that any endorsement of the placebo notion is to some degree deceptive and that placebo problems including placebo deception can be avoided by using placebo-free language. Consider the following questions from a survey of patient attitudes (Chen and Johnson 2009) that found a general lack of patient understanding of the placebo effect:

> All standard treatments have failed with a patient. Should a doctor consider it acceptable to use a placebo describing it as a "new treatment, not yet on the market but known to be effective" to calm the patient?

No language is purely neutral, so there is no ideal question, no way to avoid misleading some people. But this question uses the word placebo and suggests compounding the lie that heals with another lie about it being new treatment. The question also does not mention whether all standard treatments have failed for a dying elderly cancer patient or for a child's common fever. Not surprisingly, more than two thirds of respondents deemed this abstract situation, applicable to any patient they imagined, to be inappropriate. The answers might have been different if the question were phrased:

> Should a doctor consider it acceptable to give the following treatment (which is also explained to the patient as): a treatment that has been tried on many patients but only helps some of them, and that is unlikely to have serious harmful effects although none of its actions are fully understood.

No bothersome placebo effects to explain here, and what is here applies to everyday experience with medicine, much like the following survey question:

> Should a doctor consider putting a bandage on a painful area (especially of a child) to reduce both pain and anxiety, even if this bandage will have little known direct effect on the injury.

This action was deemed by a large majority of respondents to be appropriate. Again the response is not surprising given the everyday experiences of parents and children. Lives are not at stake here. Although the question avoids the use of the word placebo, it retains the notion of cause and effect. Since physicians and philosophers have yet to solve the puzzles of causation in medicine, the average patient cannot be expected to distinguish direct and indirect effects of bandages without some help.

The following question is framed in standard placebo terms:

> Would you be willing to take part in a placebo-controlled trial?

Fifty-nine percent of respondents said they would be willing. But what kind of placebo-controlled trial are they thinking about? The question does not say. Presumably what respondents imagine about a placebo-controlled trial depends on their general knowledge and familiarity with clinical trials. It's unlikely that respondents who would not take part were desperately seeking something that works and were imagining that they would be paid to participate in a crossover trial in which they would receive all treatments including the new drug that they hope will end their suffering.

The survey results suggest that some may have feared that they would be untreated while others believed placebos might help. We cannot assume everyone knows that some patients in the placebo group get better and some in the new drug group do not. We don't know what their answers would have been if they had been asked:

> Would you be willing to take part in a trial that compares new drug treatment with simulated drug treatment? Both

treatments have been followed by improvement in some patients.

Or perhaps:

Would you be willing to take part in an experiment in which you will receive various treatments, ranging from full-strength drugs to reduced-strength and non-drug treatments, some with more side effects and some with fewer side effects?

Again the more we can talk directly, rather than in placebo mysteries, the better. Similar considerations apply to patient consent. Instead of informing patients that they could be given the new treatment or placebo or be on a waiting list, one possibility is to say they could receive a range from the new treatment to simulated treatment to no treatment. Explain why testing something other than the new treatment is important for comparison. The notion of placebo isn't needed for patient consent. Indeed, using the problematic placebo notion that nobody fully understands interferes with consent. People are aware that the method of treatment itself, and the people who give the treatment, together with the ingredients of the treatment, can all help or harm. They can distinguish these aspects of treatment without resorting to the notion of placebo, just as we no longer resort to notions of unbalanced humors in order to explain treatments to patients.

Lies and deception after placebo

A romantic comedy film released in 2009, *The Invention of Lying,* creates an imaginary world in which nobody tells lies. In one scene the main character rushes to visit his mother who is recovering in a hospital bed after a heart attack. The doctor appears briefly, predicts that she will die that night, and honestly says that he wishes he felt something but doesn't. He laments that he does this so often that it's hardened him to suffering. He also reveals that he's in a hurry because it's fajita night at the cafeteria downstairs. He rushes off leaving the dying patient and her son to suffer the slings and arrows of outrageous comedy and of his uncensored stream-of-consciousness honesty. Fortunately for patients, our world includes medical untruths.

Clinical medicine throughout history has seen lies, deceptions, evasions, misrepresentations, exaggerations, obfuscations, omissions, understatements, concealments, negligence, fraud and many other shades of untruth, as in society in general (Sokol 2006, 2007). Lies, white and black and every shade in between, span a range of contexts, from deliberately telling a dying patient that she's doing well, to presenting the everyday smiling facade that disguises underlying anger.

Parties to lies in medicine may be anyone, including oneself. Patients lie to doctors. Doctors lie to patients. Doctors lie to doctors. Patients and doctors lie to themselves. Patients have conflicting impulses about lying, wanting to communicate yet wanting to avoid embarrassment and often wanting to please their providers. Providers in turn want to please their patients but providers have conflicting rules about lying since they are obligated to be honest but also are not allowed to tell everything they know. They have various restrictions on blunt honesty that non-professionals do not have, such as those relating to privacy and confidentiality of patient information. No single rule applies for all people in all situations, such as do not lie or deceive, do tell the truth, the whole truth and nothing but the truth.

In the context of placebo, ethical questions cannot be resolved by simply outlawing lies and deception or by making honesty mandatory. On the contrary, according to Beecher (1970), use of placebo and deceit in clinical practice is implied in the physician-patient relationship: "When a patient comes to a doctor for relief, he gives, in the act of coming, his consent to reasonable efforts to relieve him. The physician may very properly wish to pit a drug the patient has been receiving against a placebo, to see if the drug has any specific value. This is in the patient's interest. The information cannot be obtained in any other way, and the temporary deceit is acceptable." Beecher goes on to justify placebo deception on the ground that placebos may have fewer side effects than more powerful therapeutic agents. To demand no lies or deception in medicine is not workable without trivializing any notions of lying and deception. Lying cannot simply be redefined to refer only to unethical practice, for that would merely shift the question from what is lying to what is unethical.

Say a patient in a clinical trial takes a pill, reports improvement and later finds that the pill contained only sugar; that is, it's the typical placebo composed of fake medicine that apparently has a real effect. That is a kind of fakery but depending on the information provided to the patient, perhaps on a consent form authorizing use of placebos, the anticipated fakery may not be deception. Another description of placebo is real medicine that is used under false pretenses. For instance, a patient demands antibiotics for a viral infection so the physician prescribes antibiotics to please the patient, despite the ineffectiveness of antibiotics for treatment of viral infection, and the patient reports being pleased with the cure. That may be deception if the patient is led to believe that antibiotics do work against viruses.

These are different kinds of fakery and deception. The extension of placebo effects to include placebo-related effects in the absence of placebos adds another kind of deception, a sort of deception by omission; in open-hidden experiments some participants are given information about the treatment that others do not have. Again nothing is gained by putting different situations involving medical fakery and deception in the placebo category. It isn't worth the effort to put them in the placebo box then try to pull them out to untangle and explain them.

In her frequently-cited book on lying, Sissela Bok (1978) says that while physicians cannot tell the whole truth to their patients, the decision remains whether to lie and what to say. She considers the placebo to be a kind of white lie, which she takes to be, "a falsehood not meant to injure anyone, and of little moral import." Although an individual white lie may appear trivial, Bok considers the aggregate costs and harms of placebos. For instance, a patient who learns that a physician has deceptively prescribed a placebo may feel betrayed. Having listed various undesirable qualities of placebos, Bok concludes, however, "This is not to say that all placebos must be ruled out: merely that they cannot be excused as innocuous. They should be prescribed but rarely, and only after a careful diagnosis and consideration of non-deceptive alternatives; they should be used in experimentation only after subjects have consented to their use." She adds, "In a few cases, placebos may be the only reasonable alternative." Questions about lying and deception in relation to placebo must inevitably address shades of untruth, honesty, deception, lying, misstatement and variations in circumstances.

The aim of this discussion is not to adjudicate the ethical use of placebos, however, but to move from those examples of the present placebo paradigm to what may be said without the placebo notion.

Deceptive viewpoint

The self in biomedicine is often conceptually restricted to the self-correcting nature of living organisms, the physical, chemical and electrical systems that maintain life. Those biosystems are separated from the self experienced at the level of personal meaning at which placebo is said to operate.

There is a wide gulf between the account of the patient who experiences less pain after swallowing a dummy sugar pill and what is written in the pharmacology textbook that says acetylsalicylic acid will relieve pain but does not say sugar will. Aspirin and sugar are found under different headings in textbooks. The drug has an active ingredient, the claimed cause of the cure, while the placebo does not. The biomedical explanation is in terms of active ingredient where active ingredient is a proxy for a particular causal view that deems the activity to be in the ingredient. The active ingredient is a selected factor within a particular biomedical system selected for explanation.

How are some factors selected and deemed to matter more than myriad others? Clinicians and researchers are not required to inform patients or experimental subjects about many other explanatory factors beyond the scope of the active ingredient which is deemed to be the significant factor. But other factors, such as the history of the treatment, may be relevant. Every new treatment has a life cycle with varying effectiveness from discovery through initial use to widespread acceptance or rejection. Perhaps at the time a patient is offered the treatment, comparatively few people have ever received it. The historical trajectory, however, is not ordinarily deemed to be a crucial factor when considering deception, so patients don't have to be told how many people have previously been treated, what happened to them in general terms or what the specific outcomes were. Also relevant may be whether the physician is competent, perhaps having received low grades in medical school or, while having been at the top of the class, not having had time since graduation to keep up with the literature. Disclosing the physician's or the treatment's past is not viewed in biomedicine the same way as disclosing that a pill may contain only sugar.

Nor is language typically deemed to be an explanatory factor in biomedicine yet clearly language can be deliberately structured to influence the outcome. Consider this example selected from an extensive literature on medical communication: for some patients, to say "watchful waiting" has a positive connotation, while for others it is equivalent to saying they can expect no treatment; a different expectation may arise than if the phrase "active monitoring" is used (Evans et al. 2006). Is such a deliberate change in terminology a form of deception? Is there an obligation to inform the patient that what is being said may be propaganda? These and many other factors, not just the active or inactive ingredients, may be highly relevant to the success of the intervention.

Seen in light of an infinite number of explanatory factors such as these, it is curious that informing patients about the distinction between deemed active ingredients and inactive placebos matters more than information about physicians themselves, or about the known population of humans who have ever received the treatment, or the dangers of misleading language, among many other possibilities.

Language, imagery and indeed all forms of communication are subject to multiple uses and interpretations, including deceptive ones. For instance, patients in hospitals for obvious reasons tend to be sicker than people elsewhere. Yet the name of the hospital might be Metro Health Center which deceptively suggests that it's a center of health, rather than the more accurate Metro Sickness Center. Clearly the name Health Center is intended to generate healthful images associated with positive outcomes. Is this hospital's name therefore a placebo? Or consider the new medical graduate, first day on the job, who knows what unsuspecting patients do not know, that their doctor doesn't have all of the experience they believe attaches to the title of Doctor. Say this new doctor offers full disclosure, by telling every patient, "It's my first day on the job." Would they grasp the significance or remain deceived, perhaps by the title and white coat, about the doctor's powers? Would they be better off or would they worry? Perhaps some would be more confident if their new doctor were also more confident yet less forthcoming.

Deception in relation to placebo refers only to some bending of truth. Deciding where the line is, and adjudicating what is outside the line and what gets in, again illustrates the difficulty of dividing the world into placebos and non-placebos.

Placebo-free laws

Policy-makers and regulators weave placebo thinking into the social fabric by making rules for placebo use in research and against placebo use in practice. Placebo has been engrained explicitly or implicitly into medical texts, research literature, practice guidelines and legislation, with mutual reinforcement between the medical thinking that informs the rules and the rule-making that mandates medical research and practice.

In the legal realm, law professor Anup Malani (2008) explores implications of the placebo, calling for explicit legal recognition of the power of placebo. According to Malani, legal recognition of placebo effects would allow a company accused of selling a fake health product to defend itself on the grounds that the product produces placebo effects. This proposal along with other innovative ideas provides material for debate but is still deeply tied to the current notion that placebo effects exist and are powerful.

How does Malani determine the existence of placebo effects? He appears to succumb to the fallacy that the more popular a viewpoint is, the more likely it is to be true: "As a threshold matter, the sheer quantity of studies finding evidence consistent with such placebo effects makes it hard to deny they exist." Such community standards in legal contexts may protect individual experts from malpractice claims but not from generally accepted but questionable notions. That the evidence is most popularly construed in terms of placebo does not validate the paradigm. If most experts still believed in four humors then by the same threshold the effects of humoral imbalances would exist. Before the era of William Harvey, a poll of most authorities would have associated blood with heat, not with circulation. Unlike in law and politics where majority votes among justices and electors count, if the sheer quantity of scientific studies held sway, that would be the end of science as we know it. In science, the quantity of studies sometimes matters, as in the sense that one dissenting vote can carry the day if it disproves what the majority claims, and in the sense that old ideas may linger until the number of dissenters increases and the new paradigm becomes the majority view.

Malani also subscribes to a distinction between pure placebos and impure placebos that have pharmacological effects. Or to put it the other way around, they would be pharmacologically effective treatments that also have placebo effects, if indeed placebo effects could somehow be isolated from pharmacological effects. So he is forced to try to find regulatory distinctions between them while at the same time acknowledging that what he calls pure placebos might not even exist. Placebo in law cannot make more sense than placebo in medicine.

If placebo were to be replaced by a more direct approach, placebo would no longer be an acceptable explanation. To say the patient improved because of the placebo effect of a fake health product would be considered nonsense.

Placebo-free guidelines

Principles stated in various guidelines govern the use of placebos in clinical trials. For instance, the October 2008 revision of the *World Medical Association Declaration of Helsinki - Ethical Principles for Medical Research Involving Human Subjects* states:

> The benefits, risks, burdens and effectiveness of a new intervention must be tested against those of the best current proven intervention, except in the following circumstances:
>
> The use of placebo, or no treatment, is acceptable in studies where no current proven intervention exists; or

> Where for compelling and scientifically sound methodological reasons the use of placebo is necessary to determine the efficacy or safety of an intervention

> and the patients who receive placebo or no treatment will not be subject to any risk of serious or irreversible harm.

> Extreme care must be taken to avoid abuse of this option.

It's not easy to draft these contentious sorts of clauses, and the many revisions to this declaration are evidence of its problematic and actively debated nature. A general legal principle for drafting weighty documents, such as laws, regulations, and contracts, is that the presence of specific language in one part implies that the same specific language does not apply elsewhere in the document. For if the language applies generally throughout the document, then there is no reason to limit that language to only one specific part. So the reminder at the end of the quoted passage to avoid abuse seems to suggest that one should only take extreme care to avoid abuse of that option. Why not take extreme care to avoid every kind of abuse? The first part could say: take extreme care and ensure that no better alternative exists before using placebo or no treatment. Or in pursuit of medicine after placebo: take extreme care to avoid using the outdated notion of placebo.

Now let's remove the placebo language altogether, including the debated terms effectiveness and efficacy that in part depend on placebo language, and move to a general clause, applicable to all other clauses, the specific reminder to take extreme care, so that we might now debate this version:

> A new intervention must be tested against the best standard intervention, except: (1) when there is no standard intervention, or (2) if there is no risk of serious or irreversible harm and for compelling and scientifically sound methodological reasons,

a new intervention may be compared with no intervention or an intervention intended to influence the patient's beliefs, hopes and expectations.

This is not to say eliminating placebo language will end debate. Far from it. There will always be argument hinging on the powers of experts and authorities to interpret the language and decide what is the current standard intervention or what are compelling reasons, and who gets the final say. Judgment cannot be eliminated by fiat. It's not perfect but this language does contemplate the sugar pill that is intended to fool the subject into believing, hoping and expecting that the intervention works. Influences other than belief, hope and expectation may also be considered, for instance learning and conditioning. The language of belief, hope and expectation may be revised or discarded for better terms, and as we change our views of them, they may again need revision.

Placebo-free regulations

Placebo language is unnecessarily embedded in regulations. For instance, the US Food and Drug Administration (FDA) enforces a regulation (21CFR314.126a) that states:

> The purpose of conducting clinical investigations of a drug is to distinguish the effect of a drug from other influences, such as spontaneous change in the course of the disease, placebo effect, or biased observation.

This language of effect, whether drug effect or placebo effect, is problematic for the reasons raised previously in this discussion. As usual, the language of drug effect parallels and supports the language of placebo effect. Moreover, within such an effect discourse, drugs have not just an effect but multiple effects, notably good and bad effects. The quoted clause cannot be fully understood without looking further in the regulation for the characteristics of "an adequate and well-controlled study" of which the first type of control recognized is placebo concurrent control:

> Placebo concurrent control. The test drug is compared with an inactive preparation designed to resemble the test drug as far as possible. A placebo-controlled study may include additional treatment groups, such as an active treatment control or a dose-comparison control, and usually includes randomization and blinding of patients or investigators, or both.

With apologies in advance to those legislative drafters who will no doubt do a better job in regulating medicine after placebo, here is an attempt to redraft the regulation, not as a definitive version but only to show the possibilities:

> The purpose of clinical investigations is to compare the safety and effectiveness of a drug or procedure with reasonable alternatives appropriate in the circumstances.

This version replaces language of effect with language of comparison and reasonable judgment. Much of law is grounded on nothing more specific than the requirement to be reasonable and what is deemed to be reasonable changes over time. Further refinements could provide examples of appropriate alternatives that in any event would have to be justified. Here would be an opportunity to consider how reasonable are the currently unregulated controls now called placebo controls. Since there is no placebo control in medicine after placebo, there is no need to define placebo control, so the recognized types of control could amplify parts such as the manipulation of belief and expectation:

Recognized types of control depend on the aims and methodology of the investigation. One study design might compare the test drug with a simulated comparator intended to make all participants indifferent about treatment allocation. In that case evidence is required that the simulation could and did succeed. Another study design might use only the test drug but give the test group and control group different information. In that case detailed protocols for communicating among participants are required.

Further stipulations about simulated comparators could be made as study designs evolve. The reference to participant indifference highlights the typical situation, in what is now called a placebo-controlled trial, in which participants are not supposed to have any particular interest or concern one way or the other about treatment allocation.

Placebo-free medical training

Eliminating placebo from medical training may turn out to be relatively easy, since medical students apparently learn little about placebo and placebo effects from their textbooks or lectures (Raz and Guindi 2008, Bok 1974). In their formative years, medical student training about placebo is distinctly informal. After all, the current biomedical stance assures them that what does the work in medical interventions are the physical and chemical processes, based on science and technology, such as drug ingredients and surgery, not primarily the beliefs and expectations of the participants within the environment of the medical encounter. This view is inculcated in pre-clinical training, with its emphasis on basic sciences that, while providing some of the necessary scientific conceptual tools, provides no tools for inquiring into beliefs, expectations or much else about human behavior. As only one perhaps unrepresentative example, at the time of writing this document, the largest medical school in my country has no learning objectives for what its medical undergraduates must take home about placebo and does not even have an elective course for them devoted to placebo; placebo effects are covered only briefly during pharmacology lectures and their current textbook does not mention placebo.

When the question of new courses arises in medical education, a typical answer is that medical students already have too much on their agendas. With respect to placebo-free thinking, course material would have to be added, since they currently learn so little about placebo and its problems. A more fundamental reorganization than adding a few lectures would put less emphasis on pure science and technology and add more emphasis on people.

Placebo pluralism

Pluralism has a plurality of meanings. In one sense it could refer to multiple treatment alternatives, including choice of medicines and traditions, and treatment choices within a particular kind of medicine and choices among various experts, non-experts and self-help. Pluralism in medicine has more specifically been a response to the dichotomy of orthodox versus complementary alternative medicine. Beyond multiple treatments are the broader implications of multiple beliefs and practices inherent in ethnically and culturally pluralist societies.

There is also the pluralism in viewpoint discourse outlined previously that includes participant viewpoints of patient, provider and various third party interests including families, governments and private corporations. In addition to medical pluralism is the related issue of scientific pluralism that considers alternatives to a single grand unified account of the world (Kellert et al. 2006, Dale et al. 2009). Placebo pluralism touches on all of these themes.

Placebo remains a current term in medicine despite all the problems outlined here and despite many previous predictions of its demise and calls for something better. The power of placebo terminology rivals its purported power over patients. The theory of placebo has a metaphysical capacity to grab hold of the imagination and resist theory change. But placebo is only an artifact that comes from taking a particular viewpoint. From other viewpoints, placebo and placebo effects disappear.

Strong, weak or multiple views of placebo

I call the currently accepted placebo research program the weak view. This view recognizes that placebo is a problem, but supports the engrained placebo construct as if it is merely another solvable puzzle like any other scientific problem we're working on.

The more radical view proposed here, extending previous calls for the demise of placebo, is that the placebo construct cannot be fixed. It's not just a scientific problem. More evidence is not the answer. What we now associate with placebo would be better left to medical history. In this strong view, everything now associated with placebo would be better conceived in other ways. Most placebo phenomena can be better expressed using other models and language, including simply acknowledging our lack of knowledge.

We should also avoid our natural tendency to construct false opposites, as I have just done by contrasting the received view with this stronger more radical view. Other views also exist, including the possibility of pluralism in placebo viewpoints, that may lead the way to the eventual elimination of placebo language from medical practice and research. Medical researchers who do not deal directly with patients have particular views of placebo, while clinical practitioners who treat patients have their own views and patients who just want to get better have yet other views, and they can all stop saying placebo. Medicine incorporating many models is likely to be more vigorous than any single-model medicine (Nunn 2012).

Bottom line

If nothing else, try to avoid saying placebo for a while and see what creative changes may follow.

12 Extra Credit: Placebo Puzzles

Many references to paradoxes, puzzles, enigmas, contradictions and ironies appear in the placebo literature and throughout this discussion. Nobody has collected them in a convenient list, as far as I know. What follows is not an exhaustive list of placebo puzzles and paradoxes, however. On the contrary, I hope to inspire the hunt for more. I construe items in this list broadly to include that which is contrary to expectation, or beyond belief, or just puzzling, ironic or surprising and that helps to delimit the problematic placebo concept. Although the word paradox is commonly used in relation to placebo, nothing in this discussion turns on that label. Whatever word aptly describes them, I will have achieved my objective if the items in the following list shake your confidence in the notion of placebo.

Placebo definition paradoxes

One paradox noted throughout this discussion lurks in the definition of placebo as something inert that has an effect. Or something effective that is inert. That doesn't seem to make sense of either the word inert or the word effective. Finding a medically inert substance is something like the alchemist's quest for the universal solvent or the immovable object. Similarly, to define a placebo as something with non-specific effects seems strange. If you can't specify the effects, then how do you know what they are? On the other hand, if you can specify the effects, then they're specific effects.

Placebo standards paradox

As Beatrice Golomb (1995) notes, "It is paradoxical that there is no standard of evidence to support the standard of evidence." Published reports routinely fail to disclose the composition of placebo treatments (Golomb et al. 2010). Although experimenters go to great lengths to eliminate bias in drug testing, there's a loophole for the placebo that has no standards of its own.

Moral and ethical placebo paradoxes

Paradoxes also appear in moral and ethical concerns about placebos. A major ethical question, and the source of much debate, is whether placebos should be used at all, since those who get the placebo may be deprived of other treatments. A goal in clinical trials is to reduce the number of participants who get ineffective treatment, and, not incidentally, to reduce the cost of trials. One route is simply not to use a placebo but instead to do an active trial comparing two active treatments. But the distinction between placebo controls and active controls rests on shaky ground. When two active treatments are compared in the absence of placebo, both treatment groups may have similar outcomes, but there is no way to know whether either treatment is more effective in these groups than placebo.

Paradox of power

Leon (2002) has pointed out a Paradox of Power in these circumstances. The difference between two active drugs is likely to be smaller than the difference between an active drug and a placebo (or conversely, if the effect size is extremely large then a trial will not be needed to demonstrate a difference). More participants are needed to detect a small difference than a large difference. Bigger trials using active drugs mean more participants on the losing side of the experiment, more people who don't get better and who do get adverse effects. So avoiding placebos can actually result in the very problems attributed to using placebos. This paradox is part of the general ethical question of the extent to which resources should be devoted to a proliferation of competing drug brands.

Blinding binds

Philip's Paradox represents a challenge to blinding or masking in clinical trials (Ney 1986). The more potent the intervention, the more likely that participants will guess who got what treatment and the more difficult it is to claim that the trial actually was blind. The results are more methodologically successful when the experimental treatment is less successful at beating the dummy treatment. Can this paradox be avoided by comparing a treatment with no treatment instead of comparing treatment with placebo? No, then we're into the No Treatment Paradox and the different expectations associated with no treatment compared to an active treatment or to the untested person on the street.

A related irony is that, for good reason, pharmaceutical companies tout products that have fewer side effects. But treatments with more side effects are often the ones that work better at their primary target, with the side effects coming along as collateral damage. In clinical trials, active controls with apparent side effects that induce the belief and expectation that they are more effective may be more effective.

No treatment paradox

The No Treatment Paradox addresses the laudable but impossible goal of comparing placebo treatment with no treatment in a clinical trial. No treatment is not the same as doing nothing. Any ethical trial will have some contact with and influence on people receiving no treatment. The paradox does not disappear if one merely declares that the no-treatment group may not have been greatly influenced.

Efficacy-effectiveness paradox

The Efficacy-Effectiveness Paradox concerns the difference between what works for participants in clinical trials, termed efficacy, and what works for actual patients in clinical practice, termed effectiveness. The more tightly controlled the trials, the less representative they are of clinical practice. Paradoxically, clinicians try to increase what they believe is the placebo effect while in clinical trials the placebo effect is something to be minimized like noise interfering with music. For those who think placebos are noise, and only specific non-placebo effects are legitimate music, the logic is that the treatment must be louder than mere noise. For those who want to use the placebo effect itself in clinical practice, the noise of the placebo is music (Ernst 2007, Walach 2001).

Individual group irony

The Individual Group Irony is not limited to placebo-controlled trials but is inherent in the statistical approach of biomedical science. Clinicians treat individual patients. It is ironic that groups in clinical trials are measured to provide knowledge about treatments for individuals. Knowledge about other people in other circumstances is the basis for treating this individual in these circumstances.

Comorbidity paradox

Experiments are often designed to test one treatment for one disease. Typical patients, on the other hand, more likely have multiple problems and receive multiple treatments. If relatively healthy patients using only the experimental treatment are the subjects of clinical trials, then the experimental treatment's effects may be overestimated. But if typical patients with many diseases are included in clinical trials, the experimental results may be intractable.

Mystery or ignorance paradox

Consider the empowered patient who wants to be a partner with the physician, not a passive recipient of medical paternalism. The patient is primed with knowledge after searching online, talking to friends, seeking every opinion, hoping to distinguish quackery from efficacy. Has this informed patient, by trying to penetrate the mystery, foreclosed the opportunity to benefit from belief and expectation? Knowing spoils the experience, like reading a review that gives away the plot. The more mystery, the more ritual, the less questioning or searching for evidence, apparently the more powerful the magic. Questions make the illusion collapse. As Hans Christian Andersen demonstrated long ago in a different context, if it weren't for a child's questions, the Emperor would still be fully naked. To ask if the Emperor has clothes is to remove them. More than that, not to see the invisible clothes is to prove that one is too ignorant to see what everyone else pretends to see.

A physician who inspires trust may have better results but a fully trusting patient has little motivation to ask questions or seek another opinion. Ignorance need not be restricted to patients. Willful ignorance in physicians may violate various rules, including legal and moral obligations to be competent, but those are additional issues that do not change the fact that, paradoxically, ignorance can be powerful.

Enthusiasm paradox

The more enthusiasm surrounding a treatment, the more likely it is to appear to work. Conversely lack of enthusiasm can weaken the magic. But enthusiasm, like trust, is also likely to be accompanied by less desire to scrutinize the basis for the enthusiasm. Enthusiasm and skepticism are sleepless bedfellows. The enthusiast shouts, it works! The skeptic wonders how and why it works. The enthusiast says ours is not to reason why. Who cares why it works? If it helps the patient, that's the important thing! Knowledge for the enthusiast is secondary. This is not a paradox only of belief, or even of strength of belief. This is not just about reasons. The enthusiast and the skeptic may both believe that the treatment works sometimes. But they have different emotional temperatures and viewpoints. Say they agree with Beecher that it works for about one person in three. The enthusiast sees the one person who gets better while the skeptic sees the other two who don't. Enthusiasm and optimism, in addition to belief and knowledge, may influence whether the patient is in the fortunate third or the less fortunate majority.

Purposeful placebo paradox

This paradox focuses attention neither on the physician nor on the patient but on those who exhort physicians to use the powerful placebo on the basis that it could be much less trouble and would be much less expensive than active remedies. According to this view, the Emperor should continue to model his invisible fashions for the benefit of those who can see them. All that matters is that the treatment works for some patients. But here's the paradox: if you urge physicians to use the placebo because you believe it works, then you don't believe it is inert. So then how can you call it a placebo? Or if you prefer to call it a placebo because the mechanism is unknown, then how does that differ from other interventions with unknown mechanisms (which includes much of medicine) that are not called placebos?

Or suppose you prefer a different definition of placebo, not based on being inert but on being non-specific. Say we accept Evans's (2005) hypothesis that placebos are most useful for conditions related to the immune response, such as pain and swelling, and placebos can deliberately be made more effective with strong doctor patient relationships, rituals, touching, and various other known inducements. If you urge physicians to use a placebo for its specific power over specific conditions known to respond to placebos, then you have turned the non-specific remedy into something specific.

Honesty paradox

Honesty may not be the best policy but instead may be harmful, turning what has been considered placebo into nocebo. Consider only one example from the many reported cases and ethical reviews of truth-telling by doctors to patients. Speigel (1997) relates a story about the renowned advocate of the biopsychosocial medical model, George Engel, who was asked by a cancer patient whether she had male or female cancer, because she was told that male cancer is more painful. Engel replied, "You have a female cancer." Spiegel says of this story that Engel responded compassionately for therapeutic effect and healing, whereas:

> With the conviction of the mainstream biomedical paradigm prevalent today, it would be tempting to say to Dr. Engel's patient: "That question is nonsense. Cancer pain is not classified as 'male' or 'female'. Pain varies with location in the body and other factors." This response is technically honest but, in effect, it would have the impact of a nocebo. It would impair the patient's hope and morale. The doctor's honesty and conviction would serve as blinders to the patient's suffering. This type of honest statement results in a diminished sense of responsibility for the patient's well-being.

Not all patients would so readily dismiss honesty in this case as nocebo. A cancer patient commenting on this story said she thought perpetuating the lie about female cancer was the easiest response but not the best. She was concerned that he had usurped her right to know. She asked if she couldn't rely on her doctor to tell her the truth about her cancer, that it was neither male nor female, then who else could she trust? The point is not to debate issues of truth-telling in medicine but rather to say that conceiving of this story in terms of placebo or nocebo does nothing.

Placebo expertise paradox

Evidence-based medicine shifts the focus from the physician's personal experience and expertise to the impersonal statistical averages reported in medical journals. Increasing reliance on technology and specialization also limits the role of the individual physician, "Yet it is paradoxical that the more powerless the individual physician becomes, the louder the clamor for family physicians, for guides, for friends" (Spiro 1986).

If medical experts were generally known to study and use placebos, would they still be considered medical experts? Or just professional guides and friends? Consider the position of a professor at a medical school who studies placebos and teaches physicians to use them to fool patients in clinical practice. In what is their expertise? Deception? Magic? Persuasion? Friendship? The Placebo Expertise Paradox challenges physicians to assess how much of medicine is science and how much is magic. For instance Buckman and Sabbagh (1993) conclude that "Diseases need medicine, but human beings who suffer will always need a touch of magic."

Placebo career and funding paradox

Hoffer (2003) puts the question in the form of a career choice: "What bright young researcher would choose to devote a scientific career to confirming the inefficacy of implausible treatments?" In a similar vein, Ernst (2009) notes that, "...CAM research is not generally considered to be a wise career move: trained researchers from other fields have little impetus to go into CAM research, as it is neither well funded nor academically rewarding." Paradoxically, although placebo has been hailed as cheap or free medicine that deserves more research, that very fact limits research.

Unpredictability paradox

A curious thing about controlled clinical trials is that the element of chance is deliberately added. Participants are randomly assigned to the experimental intervention or control group, in the hope that uncontrolled factors will be evenly distributed and, together with blinding, so nobody can put participants in a particular group (although critics such as Worrall 2007 reject these and other reasons for randomizing). The uncertainty of randomness is used to make the results less certainly biased. Kunz and Oxman (1998) frame this paradox in these terms, "It is a paradox that unpredictability is introduced into the design of clinical trials by using random allocation to protect against the unpredictability of the extent of bias in the results of non-randomised clinical trials." The problem is also one of controllability as the other side of predictability.

Placebo permission paradox

This paradox comes from an evolutionary view of placebos. Although humans are self-organizing organisms, placebos demonstrate a need for external influences to effect internal repair. "Why should it be that we so often need what amounts to *outside permission* before taking charge of healing our own bodies?" (Humphrey 2002). This paradox or puzzle is for those who do not challenge the very existence of placebos but accept that placebos exist, are external influences and have effects. On the other hand, it may not be possible to separate internal mechanisms that may be at work, always or at any time, from specific external influences.

Suggestion paradox

Proposed explanations for placebo, such as suggestion, raise their own paradoxes. The concept of suggestion itself rests on paradoxical ground:

> Here is the paradox of suggestion: how can you induce someone to become passive (suggestible) if this passivity requires his prior acceptance? If he accepts, it is because he was already willing. But if he was willing, can we say that he passively executed a suggestion? (Borch-Jacobsen 2009).

Clearly there's more or less to the mystery of placebo than merely substituting one paradox for another, suggestion power for placebo power.

Placebo illusion

These paradoxes, or this paradox if you accept that they all stem from a concept that itself is paradoxical, ultimately go to the fundamentals of the skeptical attitude of science and the evidence-based view of medicine as compared to other accepting, believing, enthusiastic, faithful and trusting attitudes. The more faith, emotion and belief, the less science, reasoning and evidence, the more life placebo seems to have. That is the case at least for those who believe in placebo. For those of us who say placebo is an illusion, the invisible cloth is perfectly clear (Nunn 2009).

Bibliography

Allan LG, Siegel S 2002. A Signal Detection Theory Analysis of the Placebo Effect. Eval Health Prof 25: 410-20

Astbury B, Leeuw FL 2010. Unpacking Black Boxes: Mechanisms and Theory Building in Evaluation. American J. of Evaluation 31: 363

Aviram A 2006. The placebo effect of law: Law's role in manipulating perceptions. George Washington Law Review 75 (1): 54-104

Bakal D 1999. Minding the Body NY: The Guilford Press

Banerjee S 2010. Urban legend of digital drugs sweeping the Internet. Globe and Mail. July 27, 2010

Bausell RB 2007. Snake Oil Science: The Truth about Complementary and Alternative Medicine, Oxford University Press

Beecher HK 1955. The powerful placebo. JAMA 159: 1602-6

Beecher HK 1970. Research and the Individual: Human Studies. Boston: Little, Brown and Company

Beedie CJ 2007. Placebo effects in competitive sport: Qualitative data. Journal of Sports Science and Medicine 6: 21-28

Benedetti F, Arduino C, Costa S et al. 2006. Loss of expectation-related mechanisms in Alzheimer's disease makes analgesic therapies less effective. Pain 121: 133–144

Benedetti F 2007. What do you expect from this treatment? Changing our mind about clinical trials. Pain 128: 193–194

Benedetti F, Pollo A, Colloca L 2007. Opioid-Mediated Placebo Responses Boost Pain Endurance and Physical Performance: Is It Doping in Sport Competitions? The Journal of Neuroscience 27(44): 11934-11939

Benedetti F 2008. Mechanisms of placebo and placebo-related effects across diseases and treatments Annual Review of Pharmacology and Toxicology 48:33-60

Benedetti F 2009. Placebo Effects: understanding the mechanisms in health and disease. Oxford University Press

Benedetti F, Maggi G, Lopiano L, et al. 2003. Open versus hidden medical treatments: The patient's knowledge about a therapy affects the therapy outcome. Prev. Treat. 6(1)

Benedetti F, Calino E, Pollo A 2010. How Placebos Change the Patient's Brain. Neuropsychopharmacology Reviews 1–16

Bingel U, Wanigasekera V, Wiech K et al. 2011. The Effect of Treatment Expectation on Drug Efficacy: Imaging the Analgesic Benefit of the Opioid Remifentanil. Sci Transl Med 16(3): 70ra14

Bok S 1974. The Ethics of Giving Placebos. Sci Am 231(5): 17-23

Bok S 1978. Lying: Moral Choice in Public and Private Life. New York: Pantheon Books

Borch-Jacobsen M 2009. Making Minds and Madness: From Hysteria to Depression. Cambridge University Press

Borgerson K 2005. Evidence-based alternative medicine? Perspectives in Biology and Medicine 48(4): 502-515

Benson H, Friedman R 1996. Harnessing the power of the placebo effect and renaming it "remembered wellness" Annual Review of Medicine 47: 193-199

Boorse C 1976. What a Theory of Mental Health Should Be. Journal of the Theory of Social Behavior 6: 61-84

Boorse C 1977. Health as a theoretical concept. Philosophy of Science. 44: 542–73

Branthwaite A 2002. Investigating the power of imagery in marketing communication: evidence-based techniques. Qualitative Market Research 5(3): 164-171

Brody H 1980. Placebos and the Philosophy of Medicine. University of Chicago Press

Brody H 1983. Does disease have a natural history? Medical Anthropology Quarterly 14 (4):19-22

Brody H 1985. Placebo effect: an examination of Grünbaum's definition. Placebo Theory, Research and Mechanisms. White L, Tursky B, Schwartz GE (eds.) New York: The Guilford Press

Brody H 1987. Stories of Sickness. New Haven: Yale University Press

Brody H 1997. The Doctor as Therapeutic Agent. In The Placebo Effect: An Interdisciplinary Exploration. Harrington A (ed.) pp. 77-92. Cambridge, MA: Harvard University Press

Buckman R, Sabbagh K 1993. Magic or Medicine: An Investigation Of Healing & Healers, Toronto: Key Porter Books Ltd

Bunge M 2004. How Does It Work? The Search for Explanatory Mechanisms. Philosophy of the Social Sciences 34 (2): 182-210

Campbell A, Jack T, Cameron E 1991. Reticulum Cell Sarcoma: Two Complete 'Spontaneous' Regressions, in Reponse to High-Dose Ascorbic Acid Therapy. Oncology 48: 495-497

Campos DG 2011. On the distinction between Peirce's abduction and Lipton's Inference to the best explanation. Synthese 180: 419–442

Caspi O, Bootzin RR 2002. Evaluating How Placebos Produce Change: Logical and Causal Traps and Understanding Cognitive Explanatory Mechanisms. Evaluation & the Health Professions 25(4): 436-464

Cassell EJ 1982. The nature of suffering and the goals of medicine. New England Journal of Medicine 306: 639-645

Cassell EJ 2004. The Nature of Suffering and the Goals of Medicine. Oxford University Press

Cartwright N 2007. Are RCTs the Gold Standard? BioSocieties 2: 11–20

Chalmers I 1998. Evidence of the effects of heathcare: a plea for a single standard across 'orthodox' and 'complementary' medicine. International Congress and Symposium Series. Royal Society of Medicine 233: 7-12

Chen G, Johnson MH 2009. Patients' attitudes to the use of placebos: results from a New Zealand survey. NZMJ 122 (296): 35-46

Cherniak PE 2010. Would the elderly be better off if they were given more placebos? Geriatr Gerontol Int 10:131–137

Clark S 1997. Thinking with Demons: The Idea of Witchcraft in Early Modern Europe. Oxford University Press

Clifford V 2011. The placebo mystique: Implications for clinical trial methodology. Journal of Paediatrics and Child Health 47: 361–366

Colloca L, Benedetti F 2005. Placebos and painkillers: is mind as real as matter? Nat Rev Neurosci 6:545-52

Colloca L, Miller FG 2011. How placebo responses are formed: a learning perspective. Phil. Trans. R. Soc. B 366: 1859–1869

Critelli JW, Neumann KF 1984. The Placebo: Conceptual Analysis of a Construct in Transition. American Psychologist 39(1) 32-39

Dale R, Dietrich E, Chemero A 2009. Explanatory Pluralism in Cognitive Science. Cognitive Science 33: 739–742

de Craen AJM, Roos PJ, de Vries AL, Kleijnen J 1996. Effect of colour of drugs: systematic review of perceived effect of drugs and of their effectiveness. BMJ 313: 1624-1626

de la Fuente-Fernández R, Stoessl JA 2002. The Biochemical Bases for Reward: Implications for the Placebo Effect. Evaluation & the Health Professions 25(4): 387-398

Delkeskamp-Hayes C, Cutter MAC (eds.) 1993. Science, Technology, and the Art of Medicine: European-American Dialogues. Dordrecht: Kluwer Academic Publishers

Della Sala S (ed.) 1999. Mind Myths: Exploring Popular Assumptions about Mind and Body. Chichester: John Wiley & Sons

Dennett DC 1978. Why you can't make a computer that feels pain. Synthese 38: 415-456

Devereaux PJ, Manns BJ et al. 2001. Blinding Terminology in Randomized Controlled Trials. JAMA 285(15): 2000-2003

Dixon B 1978. Beyond the Magic Bullet. London: George Allen & Unwin

Di Blasi Z, Harkness E, Ernst E et al 2001. Influence of context effects on health outcomes: a systematic review. Lancet 357: 757-762

Duffin J 2010. History of Medicine: a scandalously short introduction. Toronto: University of Toronto Press

Egeth M 2009. Meta-meta-placebo and -curabo: You might get better just by reading this paper. Medical Hypotheses. doi: 10.1016/j.mehy.2008.08.034

Einstein A, Infeld L 1938. The evolution of physics, the growth of ideas from early concepts to relativity and quanta. New York: Simon and Schuster

Ellison CG, Burdette AM 2011. Religion and the Sense of Control among U.S. Adults. Sociology of Religion. doi:10.1093/socrel/srr035

Enck P, Benedetti F, Schedlowski M 2008. New Insights into the Placebo and Nocebo Responses. Neuron 59: 195-206

Ernst E 2001. Towards a scientific understanding of placebo effects. In Peters D (ed.) Understanding the placebo effect in complementary medicine. Elsevier Health Sciences

Ernst E 2007. Placebo: new insights into an old enigma. Drug Discovery Today 12(9-10): 413-418

Ernst E 2009. Complementary and Alternative Medicine: between evidence and absurdity. Perspectives in Biology and Medicine 52(2): 289–303

Ernst E, Resch KL 1995. Concept of true and perceived placebo effects. BMJ 311: 551–553

Evans D 2003. Placebo: the Belief Effect, London: HarperCollins

Evans D 2005. Suppression of the acute-phase response as a biological mechanism for the placebo effect. Medical Hypotheses 64: 1–7

Evans I, Thornton H, Chalmers I 2006. Testing Treatments Better Research for Better Healthcare. (reprinted 2010) London: Pinter & Martin Ltd

Fergusson D, Glass KC, Waring D, Shapiro S 2004. Turning a blind eye: the success of blinding reported in a random sample of randomised, placebo controlled trials. BMJ 328:432

Finniss DG, Kaptchuk, TJ Franklin Miller, F, Benedetti F 2010. Biological, clinical, and ethical advances of placebo effects. Lancet 375: 686–95

Fisher RA 1935. The Design of Experiments. Edinburgh: Oliver & Boyd

Fleck L 1979. The Genesis and Development of a Scientific Fact, Trenn TJ and Merton RK (eds.) Chicago: University of Chicago Press

Golomb BA 1995. Paradox of placebo effect. Nature 375: 530

Golomb BA, Erickson LC, Koperski S et al. 2010. What's in Placebos: Who Knows? Analysis of Randomized, Controlled Trials. Annals of Internal Medicine 153(8): 532-535

Gøtzsche PC 1994. Is there logic in the placebo? Lancet 344(8927): 925-926

Gøtzsche PC 2007. Rational diagnosis and treatment: evidence-based clinical decision-making, 4th ed. Chichester: John Wiley & Sons Ltd.

Gould SJ 1991. Advertising and hypnotic suggestion: the construct of advertising suggestion. In Schumaker JF (ed.) Human Suggestibility: Advances in theory, research, and application. New York: Routledge

Grob CS, Danforth AL, Chopra GS et al. 2010. Pilot Study of Psilocybin Treatment for Anxiety in Patients With Advanced-Stage Cancer. Arch Gen Psychiatry. doi:10.1001/archgenpsychiatry.2010.116

Grünbaum A 1985. Explication and implications of the placebo concept. In

White L, Tursky B, Schwartz GE (eds.) Placebo Theory, Research, and Mechanisms, New York: The Guilford Press

Hahn RA, Kleinman A 1983. Belief as Pathogen, Belief as Medicine: "Voodoo Death" and the "Placebo Phenomenon" in Anthropological Perspective. Medical Anthropology Quarterly 14(4)3, 16-19

Hansen K, Kappel K 2010. The proper role of evidence in complementary/alternative medicine. J. Med. Philos. 35(1): 7-18

Harrington A 2006. The Many Meanings of the Placebo Effect: Where They Came From, Why They Matter. BioSocieties 1: 181193

Harrington A 2008. The Cure Within: A History of Mind-Body Medicine, New York: WW Norton & Company

Harrington A 2011. The Placebo Effect: What's Interesting for Scholars of Religion? Zygon 46(2): 265-280

Henningsen P, Zimmermann T, Sattel H 2003. Medically unexplained physical symptoms, anxiety, and depression: a meta-analytic review. Psychosomatic medicine 65(4): 528–33

Hoffer JL 2003. Complementary or alternative medicine: the need for plausibility. CMAJ 168(2): 180-182

Hill AB 1963. Medical ethics and controlled trials. BMJ 1: 1043-1049

Hill AB 1965. The environment and disease: association or causation? Proc. R. Soc. Med. 58: 295–300

Howick J 2009. Questioning the methodologic superiority of 'placebo' over 'active' controlled trials. Am. J. of Bioethics–Neuroscience 9(9): 34-48

Hróbjartsson A 1996. The uncontrollable placebo effect. European Journal of Clinical Pharmacology 50(5): 345-348

Hróbjartsson A 2008. Clinical placebo interventions are unethical, unnecessary and unprofessional. J. Clin. Ethics 19:66–9

Hróbjartsson A, Gøtzsche PC 2001. Is the Placebo Powerless? An Analysis of Clinical Trials Comparing Placebo with No Treatment. New England Journal of Medicine 344: 1594-1602

Hróbjartsson A, Gøtzsche PC 2004. Is the placebo powerless? Update of a systematic review with 52 new randomised trials comparing placebo with no treatment. J. Int. Med. 256: 91-100

Hróbjartsson A, Gøtzsche PC 2004. Placebo interventions for all clinical conditions, Updated Cochrane Review, Cochrane Database of Systematic Reviews, Issue 3, Art. No. CD003974

Hróbjartsson A, Gøtzsche PC 2010. Placebo interventions for all clinical conditions. Cochrane Database of Systematic Reviews Issue 1. Art. No. CD003974

Humphrey N 2002. Great expectations: the evolutionary psychology of faith healing and the placebo effect. In Humphrey N (ed.) The mind made flesh: essays from the frontiers of psychology and evolution. New York: Oxford University Press, 255–285

Hunter KM 1986. "There was this one guy ...": the uses of anecdotes in medicine. Perspect. Biol. Med. 29(4): 619-30

Inlow WD 1946. Medicine: Its Nature and Definition. Bulletin of the History of Medicine 19: 249-273

Ioannidis JPA 2005. Why Most Published Research Findings Are False. PLoS Med 2(8): e124. doi: 10.1371/journal.pmed.0020124

Jonas WB 2011. Reframing placebo in research and practice. Phil. Trans. R. Soc. B 366: 1896-1904

Jopling DA 2008. Talking cures and placebo effects. Oxford University Press

Kaptchuk TJ 1998. Intentional Ignorance: A History of Blind Assessment and Placebo Controls in Medicine. Bulletin of the History of Medicine 72(3): 389-433

Kaptchuk TJ 2001. The double-blind, randomized, placebo-controlled trial: Gold standard or golden calf? J. of Clinical Epidemiology 54: 541–549

Kaptchuk TJ, Kelley JM, Deykin A et al. 2008. Do "placebo responders" exist? Contemporary Clinical Trials 29: 587-595

Kaptchuk TJ, Shaw J, Kerr CE et al. 2009. "Maybe I Made Up the Whole Thing": Placebos and Patients' Experiences in a Randomized Controlled Trial. Cult. Med. Psychiatry 33: 382–411

Kaptchuk TJ, Friedlander E, Kelley JM et al. 2010. Placebos without Deception: A Randomized Controlled Trial in Irritable Bowel Syndrome. PLoS ONE 5(12): e15591. doi:10.1371/journal.pone.0015591

Kalasountas V, Reed J, Fitzpatrick J 2007. The Effect of Placebo-Induced

Changes in Expectancies on Maximal Force Production in College Students. Journal of Applied Sport Psychology 19(1): 116-124

Kellert SH, Longino HE, Waters CK (eds.) 2006. Scientific pluralism, Minnesota Studies in the Philosophy of Science (Vol. XIX). Minneapolis: University of Minnesota Press

Kienle GS, Kiene H 1997 The powerful placebo effect: Fact or fiction? J. Clin. Epidemiol. c50: 1311–1318

Kirsch I (ed.) 1999. How expectancies shape experience. Washington: American Psychological Association

Kirsch I 1999b. Hypnosis and Placebos: Response Expectancy as a Mediator of Suggestion Effects. Anales de Psicología 15(1): 99-110

Kirsch I, Weixel LJ 1988. Double-blind versus deceptive administration of a placebo. Behav. Neurosci. 102(2): 319-323

Klopfer B 1957. Psychological variables in human cancer. Journal of Projective Techniques 21(4): 330-41 In Megargee EI, Speilberger CD (eds.) 1992. Personality Assessment in America. Hillsdale: New Jersey, Lawrence Erlbaum Associates, 58-67

Koshi EB, Short CA 2007. Placebo Theory and Its Implications for Research and Clinical Practice: A Review of the Recent Literature. Pain Practice 7(1) 4–20

Kottow M 2010. The improper use of research placebos. Journal of Evaluation in Clinical Practice 16: 1041–1044

Kroger WS 1977. Clinical and experimental hypnosis in medicine, dentistry, and psychology. Philadelphia: Lippincott Company

Kunz R, Oxman AD 1998. The unpredictability paradox: review of empirical comparisons of randomised. and non-randomised clinical trials. BMJ. 317: 1185-1190

Lakoff G 1987. Women, Fire, and Dangerous Things: What Categories Reveal About the Mind. Chicago: Univ. of Chicago Press

Lamberty GJ 2008. Understanding Somatization in the Practice of Clinical Neuropsychology, New York: Oxford University Press

Langer EJ 1975. The illusion of control. Journal of Personality and Social Psychology 32(2): 311-328

Leon AC 2000. Placebo Protects Subjects From Nonresponse: A Paradox of Power. Archives of General Psychiatry 57: 329-330

Lichtenberg P, Heresco-Levy U, Nitzan U 2004. The ethics of the placebo in clinical practice. J. Med. Ethics 30:551–4

Lindahl O, Lindwall L 1982. Is all therapy just a placebo effect? Metamedicine 3: 255-259

Linde K, Witt CM, Streng A et al. 2007. The impact of patient expectations on outcomes in four randomized controlled trials of acupuncture in patients with chronic pain. Pain 128: 264–71

Louhiala P, Puustinen R 2008. Rethinking the placebo effect. Medical Humanities 34: 107-109

Louhiala P 2009. The ethics of the placebo in clinical practice revisited. J. Med. Ethics 35: 407–409

Luborsky L, Singer B, Luborsky L 1975. Comparative studies of psychotherapies: Is it true that "everyone has won and all must have prizes"? Archives of General Psychiatry 32(8): 995-1008

Luo M 2004. For Exercise in New York Futility, Push Button. New York Times February 27, 2004

Macedo A, Farrè M, Baños J 2003. Placebo effect and placebos: what are we talking about? Some conceptual and historical considerations. European Journal of Clinical Pharmacology 59(4): 337-342

Machamer P, Darden L, Craver CF 2000. Thinking about Mechanisms. Philosophy of Science 67(1): 1-25

Malani A 2008. Regulation with placebo effects. Duke Law Journal 58: 411-472

Manek NJ, Tiller WA 2011. A new perspective on "the placebo effect": Untangling the entanglement. Medical Hypotheses doi: 10.1016/j.mehy.2011.06.047

Masling JM 1997. On the Nature and Utility of Projective Tests and Objective Tests. Journal of Personality Assessment 69(2): 257-270

Meissner K, Distel H, Mitzdorf U 2007. Evidence for placebo effects on physical but not on biochemical outcome parameters: a review of clinical trials. BMC Medicine 5:3 http://www.biomedcentral.com/1741-7015/5/3

Miceli M, Castelfranchi C 2010. Hope: the power of wish and possibility. Theory & Psychology 20(2): 251–276

Milgram S 1963. Behavioral study of obedience. Journal of Abnormal and Social Psychology 67: 371–378

Miller FG, Emanuel EJ, Rosenstein DL et al. 2004. Ethical Issues Concerning Research in Complementary and Alternative Medicine. JAMA 291(5): 599-604

Miller FG, Rosenstein DL 2006. The nature and power of the placebo effect. Journal of Clinical Epidemiology 59: 331–335

Miller FG, Kaptchuk TJ 2008a. The power of context: reconceptualizing the placebo effect. J. R. Soc. Med. 101: 222–225

Miller FG, Kaptchuk TJ 2008b. Deception of Subjects in Neuroscience: An Ethical Analysis. The Journal of Neuroscience 28(19): 4841–4843

Miller FG, Colloca L, Kaptchuk TJ 2009. The Placebo Effect: Illness and Interpersonal Healing. Perspectives in Biology and Medicine 52(4): 518-39

Miller FG, Colloca L 2011. The placebo phenomenon and medical ethics: Rethinking the relationship between informed consent and risk–benefit assessment. Theor. Med. Bioeth. 32: 229–243

Moerman DE 2002a. Explanatory mechanisms for placebo effects: cultural influences and the meaning response. In The Science of the Placebo - Toward an Interdisciplinary Research Agenda. BMJ Books

Moerman DE 2002b. Medicine, meaning, and the "placebo effect" London: Cambridge University Press

Moerman DE 2003. "Placebo" versus "meaning": The case for a change in our use of language. Prevention & Treatment 6:1-5

Moll A 1891. Hypnotism. London: Walter Scott

Montgomery K 2006. How Doctors Think: Clinical Judgement and the Practice of Medicine. Oxford University Press

Moseley JB, O'Malley K, Petersen NJ et al. 2002. A controlled trial of arthroscopic surgery for osteoarthritis of the knee. New England Journal of Medicine 347:81–88

Ney PG 1986. Double blind: double talk or are there better ways to do research? Medical Hypotheses 21: 119-126

Nickerson RS 1998. Confirmation Bias: A Ubiquitous Phenomenon in Many Guises. Review of General Psychology 2(2): 175-220

Nunn R 2008. Evidence-Based Medicine and Limits to the Literature Search. Journal of Evaluation in Clinical Practice 14: 672–678

Nunn R 2009. It's time to put the placebo out of our misery. BMJ 338:b1568

Nunn R 2009b. Preparing for a Post-placebo Paradigm: ethics and choice of control in clinical trials. Am. J. of Bioethics - Neuroscience 9(9): 51-2

Nunn R 2009c. Placebo effects without placebos? More reason to abandon the paradoxical placebo. Am. J. of Bioethics - Neuroscience 9(12): 50-52

Nunn R 2012. Many Models Medicine: Diversity as the Best Medicine. Journal of Evaluation in Clinical Practice. 18: 974–978

Nwoye A 2011. Ontological Structure and Complexity of Therapeutic Hope: A Multidimensional Perspective. Psychother. Politics. Int. 9: 3–19

Orne MT 1962. On the social psychology of the psychological experiment: With particular reference to demand characteristics and their implications. American Psychologist 17: 776-783

Orne MT 2009. Demand Characteristics and the Concept of Quasi-Controls. In Rosenthal R, Rosnow RL, Artifacts in Behavioral Research: Robert Rosenthal and Ralph L Rosnow's Classic Books. Oxford University Press

Osgood CE, Suci G, Tannenbaum P 1957. The Measurement of Meaning. University of Illinois Press

Pargament KI, Cummings J 2010. Anchored by Faith: Religion as a Resilience Factor. In Reich JW, Zautra AJ, Hall JS (eds.) Handbook of Adult Resilience. New York: The Guildford Press

Park LC, Covi U 1965. Nonblind placebo trial: an exploration of neurotic patients' responses to placebo when its inert content is disclosed. Archives of General Psychiatry 12: 336-45

Papac RJ 1996. Spontaneous regression of cancer. Cancer Treatment Reviews 22: 395-423

Pellegrino ED, Thomasma DC 1981. A Philosophical Basis of Medical Practice: Toward a Philosophy and Ethic of the Healing Profession. Oxford: Oxford University Press

Peirce CS 1878. How to make our ideas clear. Popular Science Monthly 12: 286-302

Pollo A, Carlino E, Benedetti F 2011. Placebo mechanisms across different conditions: from the clinical setting to physical performance. Phil. Trans. R. Soc. B 366: 1790–1798

Raz A, Guindi D 2008. Placebos and Medical Education. MJM 11(2): 223-226

Rodin J 1986. Aging and health: effects of the sense of control. Science 233 (4770):1271-6

Rosnow RL, Rosenthal R 1997. People studying people: artifacts and ethics in behavioral research. New York: WH Freeman

Sackett DL 2007. Commentary: Measuring the success of blinding in RCTs: don't, must, can't or needn't? International Journal of Epidemiology 36:664–665

Scottish Society of Physicians 1971. Ischaemic Heart Disease: A Secondary Prevention Trial Using Clofibrate. BMJ 4: 775-784

Schulz KF, Grimes DA 2002. Blinding in randomised trials: hiding who got what. Lancet 359: 696–700

Schulz KF, Chalmers I, Altman DG 2002. The landscape and lexicon of blinding in randomized trials. Annals of Internal Medicine 136(3): 254-9

Shapiro K and Shapiro E 1997. The Powerful Placebo : From Ancient Priest to Modern Physician. Baltimore: The Johns Hopkins University Press

Sherman R, Hickner J 2007. Academic Physicians Use Placebos in Clinical Practice and Believe in the Mind–Body Connection. Journal of General Internal Medicine 23(1): 7-10

Shiv B, Carmon Z, Ariely D 2005. Placebo Effects of Marketing Actions: Consumers May Get What They Pay For. Journal of Marketing Research 42(4): 383–393

Silverman I 1968. Role-Related Behavior of Subjects in Laboratory Studies of Attitude Change. Journal of Personality and Social Psychology 8(4-1): 343-348

Sloan RP, Bagiella E, Powell T 1999. Religion, spirituality, and medicine. Lancet 353: 664–67

Sokol DK 2006. How the doctor's nose has shortened over time; a historical overview of the truth-telling debate in the doctor–patient relationship. J. R. Soc. Med. 99: 632–636

Sokol DK 2007. Can deceiving patients be morally acceptable? BMJ 334: 984-986

Solomon M 2008. Epistemological Reflections on the Art of Medicine and Narrative Medicine. Perspectives in Biology and Medicine 51(3); 406-417

Spiegel H 1997. Nocebo: The Power of Suggestibility. Preventive Medicine 26: 616–621

Spiro HM 1986. Doctors, patients and placebos, New Haven: Yale University Press

Stein HF 1983. On Placebos. To Cure, to Control, to Please: Medicine after the Demise of "The Placebo" Medical Anthropology Quarterly 15(1); 4-17

Stewart-Williams S 2004. The Placebo Puzzle: Putting Together the Pieces. Health Psychology 23(2): 198–206

Stewart-Williams S, Podd J 2004. The Placebo Effect: Dissolving the Expectancy Versus Conditioning Debate. Psychological Bulletin 130(2); 324–340

Stoker M 1980. New medicine and new biology. BMJ 281 (6256):1678–82.

Taleb NN 2007. The Black Swan: The Impact of the Highly Improbable. New York: Random House

Tang PCL 1999. The Monamine Hypothesis, Placebos, and Problems of Theory Construction in Psychology and Psychiatry. The Social Science Journal 36 (4): 595–602

Tasso A, Pérez NA 2008. Parsing everyday suggestibility: what does it tell us about hypnosis? In Nash MR, Barnier AJ (eds.) The Oxford handbook of hypnosis: theory, research and practice. Oxford University Press

Taylor SE 1989. Positive Illusions: Creative Self-Deception and the Healthy Mind. New York: Basic Books, Inc.

Thompson JJ, Ritenbaugh C, Nichter M 2009. Reconsidering the Placebo Response from a Broad Anthropological Perspective. Cult. Med. Psychiatry 33:112–152

Toulmin S 1961. Foresight and Understanding: An inquiry into the aims of Science. Bloomington: Indiana University Press

Upshur R 1997. Certainty, probability and abduction: why we should look to CS Peirce rather than Gödel for a theory of clinical reasoning. Journal for Evaluation in Clinical Practice 3(3): 201-206

van Reekum R 2010. Placebo Problems: Power and Persecution, or Paranoia? ch. 23 of When Research Goes Off the Rails: Why It Happens and What You Can Do About It. Streiner DL, Sidani S (eds.) New York: Guilford Press

Waber RL, Baba Shiv B, Ziv Carmon Z et al. 2008. Commercial Features of Placebo and Therapeutic Efficacy. JAMA 299(9): 1016-1017

Walach H 2001. The Efficacy Paradox in Randomized Controlled Trials of CAM and Elsewhere: Beware of the Placebo Trap. The Journal of Alternative and Complementary Medicine 7(3): 213-218

Wall PD 1996. The Placebo Effect, ch. 8 of Velmans M (ed.) Science of Consciousness: Psychological, Neuropsychological, and Clinical Reviews. Florence, Kentucky: Routledge

Wampold BE, Minami T, Tierney SC, et al. 2005. The placebo is powerful: Estimating placebo effects in medicine and psychotherapy from randomized clinical trials. Journal of Clinical Psychology 61: 835–854.

Weisberg DS, Keil FC, Goodstein J et al. 2008. The seductive allure of neuroscience explanations. J. Cogn. Neurosci. 20(3): 470–477

Wootton D 2006. Bad medicine: doctors doing harm since Hippocrates. Oxford University Press

Worrall J 2007. Why There's No Cause to Randomize. The British Journal for the Philosophy of Science 58(3): 451-488

Zubieta JK, Stohler CS 2009. Neurobiological mechanisms of placebo responses. Annals of the New York Academy of Sciences 1156: 198-210

About the author

Robin Nunn received a PhD from the University of Toronto and is a specialist in medical epistemology and bioethics.